AFFORDABLE HEALTH AND FITNESS

AFFORDABLE HEALTH AND FITNESS

THE BUSINESS OF HEALTH AND FITNESS

Chuck Thompson

ISBN-13: 9780692763445
ISBN-10: 0692763449
Library of Congress Control Number: 2016912663
Chuck Thompson, Jacksonville, FL

I dedicate this book to my amazing wife, Zarita "Cherry" Thompson, and my four children, Chaz, Christian, Coley, and Azha. I am truly blessed with two angels and three champions. It is because of their sacrifices and support I am able to realize my dream of making a difference in the world by helping others. Cherry has devoted her life to me and our children, giving us the joy of being members of a loving, happy family. She is just as proud of her titles of nurturer, wife, and mother as I am of mine as father, husband, and founder of MMC®. Together, we have found balance.

Cherry, I am not worthy of you, but I am eternally grateful for your love and honored to be your husband; I know I married up. Thank you for everything but most of all, thank you for saying yes. I love you baby.

Revolutionize: To change something radically—to
cause a radical change in something such
as a method or approach.
—*Encarta Dictionary*

904-217-3762
877-620-8135
chuck@mmctoday.com
chuck@chuckthompson.guru

TABLE OF CONTENTS

Introduction · xi

Chapter 1   Health Clubs in the 1980s · · · · · · · · · · · · · · · · · 1

Chapter 2   The Fitness Explosion · 29

Chapter 3   The Backbone of the Business · · · · · · · · · · · · · · 62

Chapter 4   Selling Club Memberships by the Thousands · · · · 99

Chapter 5   Marketing Essentials · 125

Chapter 6   Putting All the Pieces Together · · · · · · · · · · · · · 158

Chapter 7   The Membership That Revolutionized the
Health-Club Industry· 185

Chapter 8   On the Road Again · 213

Chapter 9   Be Careful What You Wish For· · · · · · · · · · · · · · 242

Chapter 10 Understanding the Task at Hand · · · · · · · · · · · · 271

INTRODUCTION

I n this book, I share my experiences of working in the health-club business as a young man full of ambition and testosterone in the 1980s. I engineered a health-club marketing campaign that revolutionized the health-club industry as well as the golf industry. When I first started in the business, a health-club membership was only for the upper classes; today, you can buy a membership in just about every city or town for as low as $99.00 a year or $9.99 per month. This is because the marketing campaign I engineered to engage an untapped market (consumers who had no interest in health and fitness) that is now defined as the deconditioned market (a.k.a. couch potatoes) went viral throughout the 1990s and has now (in 2016) become the norm.

Since the inception of MMC® (Mulligan Marketing Concepts®), my team and I have worked with over seven hundred membership-based businesses and raised more than a half a billion dollars in revenue for our clients while bringing affordable health and fitness to everyone in America. In total, I have been directly responsible for selling more than one million memberships and tens of millions of memberships indirectly during my thirty-five-year career. My marketing concept of using a "lost leader" (not "loss leader," which is the traditional concept; "lost leader" is a phrase I coined) partnered with a lower barrier-to-entry changed the health-club business forever.

In the 1980s, health clubs were popping up on every corner, just as Starbucks is today. By the 1990s there was too much inventory (supply) and not enough health-and-fitness-conscious consumers (demand) to support all of the new clubs. The so-called experts were throwing up their hands in bewilderment while I rolled up my sleeves. In this book, I will show you how I revolutionized the industry and reveal the necessary secrets as well as my professional sales and marketing systems so you too can make your mark with your health-and-fitness product or service.

Health clubs need new members to grow their businesses, but there are not enough health-and-fitness-conscious consumers to sustain the more than thirty-five thousand member-based fitness businesses. I designed my no-risk, self-funding campaign to target consumers who are not yet health-and-fitness conscious—a demography completely ignored by the fitness industry.

MMC® is the only company to profile consumers based on their buying patterns and spending habits for health clubs. My team looks for consumers who have purchased within the health, fitness, or diet categories but have not committed to a health-club membership. My team then prequalifies the consumer through a criteria-based formula. My goal is simple: focus on identifying, engaging, and locking up relationships with untapped markets to bring in new segments of consumers who drastically increases revenue for my clients.

Anyone in the health-club industry, whether he or she is a health-club owner, sales representative, developer, marketer, retailer, merchandiser, entrepreneur, or someone in any of the numerous other occupations within the health, fitness, wellness, spa, dietary, or nutrition industries, will find my experience and teachings extremely useful. With my help, learn how to successfully sell and promote any health-and-fitness product or service.

If you are a member of a health club, thinking about joining a health club, or wanting to lose weight but have never been able to commit to and stick with a healthy lifestyle, you need to read this book because I teach the psychological triggers that all professional trainers and fitness experts use to motivate people to take action today!

As a health-and-fitness-conscious consumer reading this book, you will learn the ins and outs of the health-club industry, acquiring the knowledge to get enormous discounts on memberships, saving yourself thousands of dollars by avoiding inflated dues and fees. If you are sedentary, you'll find the motivation in these pages to take action today and change your life forever; if you are a trainer, you will learn all of the psychological triggers necessary to motivate and encourage your clients as well as a step-by-step system to uncover your clients' and prospects' fears, goals, and unmet needs along with the very best professional sales to lock up new relationships and sell more training sessions. As an entrepreneur, you'll learn how to package, market, and professionally sell any health-and-fitness product or service; as an employee, you'll learn how to make yourself indispensable and have job security for life; and as an owner, you'll learn how to grow your business beyond your wildest imagination and put worry and fear in the past, where they belong.

I also share my opinion on the antiquated paradigms, people, and procedures that are killing the industry today. There is something in this book for everyone, because I take you on an educational journey using my thirty-five-year career in the health-club industry as a guide, and show you how I revolutionized the health-club industry, and give you the tools to penetrate new markets, engage prospects, and thrive in the greatest industry of all—health-and-fitness. Enjoy the journey.

Wishing you good health and prosperity,
Chuck Thompson

PS. Please take a few minutes and write a review for my book and post it on as many websites and platforms as possible, with a direct link to where your friends and followers can buy *Affordable Health and Fitness: The Business of Health and Fitness,* and be sure to register with my company and personal websites www.mmctoday.com, www.healthclubmarketingmmc.com and www.chuckthompson. guru (not dot com) for freebies and updates. If you wish to contact us at MMC®, you may call 904-217-3762; toll free 877-620-8135 or e-mail me at chuck@mmctoday.com. For comments or any other correspondence, please use my personal address at chuck@chuck-thompson.guru (not dot com). Thank you, and enjoy the book.

CHAPTER 1

HEALTH CLUBS IN THE 1980S

Sex, Fitness, and Rock 'n' Roll

It was 1982, and I was nineteen years old. I was contemplating going to college and majoring in business, but I needed to work and save some money. I had enrolled in a community college in Knoxville to stay on track, but I couldn't focus—my ex-girlfriend went to the same college, and although I was still in love with her, she didn't share the same feelings. It was very distracting, to say the least. My emotions, coupled with my lack of funds, drove me to drop out and get a job. Knoxville is a college town, and I was a partier, so I fit in well. I got a job in one of the student cafeterias, posed as a student, and met a lot of cool people. Although I was almost penniless (part-time work in a cafeteria doesn't pay well), I always had a place to crash and free parties to go to because during that year, I dated three girls who were students at the University of Tennessee. One lived in a dorm, one lived in an on-campus apartment, and the other lived in an apartment off campus but right across the street from the university. I was off and on with all of them, and with all girls I dated, for that matter. I loved the life of an unattached college student, and although I wasn't enrolled in any classes, I was living the college experience to the fullest.

Education has always been my top priority because I know what it is like to work with my back and earn a living with the sweat of my brow. In my adolescent years, I worked all kinds of jobs, including hauling hay, working in tobacco fields, washing dishes, delivering newspapers and groceries, cleaning horse stalls, mowing lawns, shoveling snow, and doing a bunch of other backbreaking jobs. My parents were both blue-collar workers and believed in hard work. I was determined to be the first in our family to attain a college education so I could use my brain and not my brawn to earn a living. Hard work is good for people, but I prefer to work my sixteen-hour days in air conditioning as opposed to out in the sun.

At nineteen, my interests were simple: I loved women, I loved learning, I loved listening to good rock 'n' roll, driving a nice car, and knowing I was growing intellectually. My priorities were polar opposites from those of my parents. Later in life, I discovered how important it is to understand generational differences in attitudes and behaviors, which not only helped me in my personal life but also influenced the effectiveness of my future marketing campaigns and sales systems. As I share this information with you, you will be surprised to see how profoundly that knowledge will impact the marketing strategy you choose for your products or services.

One of the girls I had been dating at UT went home to visit her family in Nashville, so I decided to follow her. I liked Nashville. It was a much larger city than Knoxville, and since I love music, I decided to stay in Music City and get a job. My first job interview was with a water-supply company, and the second was with a health club. Back then, filtered water was just entering the marketplace, and the water-supply company was willing to send me to school, pay my expenses, and provide me with a modest salary while I was in training. I could see the enormous potential of this new industry and was very excited about the opportunity. I also knew this was a job that would make my mother proud of me because of the security and benefits it offered. The desire to please her and make her happy was definitely weighing on me. I knew her preference for the job was stemmed from love and a desire for me to become financially secure, successful, and happy. Like most mothers, she wanted me to settle down, get married, have kids, and live in a house with a white picket fence.

I aced the interview at the water-supply company and was offered the job on the spot. I was very proud of this victory because normally an interview with this company was a three-tier process. The VP I interviewed with loved me; he even mentioned how impressed he was with my enthusiasm, my relevant questions, my look, as well as the fact that I had done my homework on the product and the company, and he said he knew he was choosing the best applicant for the job. I was stoked because I knew purified mineral water was going to become huge as consumers became more health conscious; it was the equivalent of entering the ground level of the dot-com industry in the 1990s. Now, I just had to go to the health club for my next interview and politely tell them I had chosen to accept another job.

I wasn't too excited about the second interview anyway. I had played some organized sports (football, basketball, and baseball), and the thought of hanging out all day with a bunch of jocks and pumping iron wasn't appealing to me at all. I had done enough of that during my school years. Besides, I had all but made up my mind I was going to take the water-sales position. It was a no-brainer. I knew sales equaled unlimited earning potential and opportunities for growth, and these were two things I wanted in life. My parents wanted me to have financial stability via a guaranteed paycheck each week, but that route came with restrictions in financial growth and limited opportunities. Sales appealed to me because I knew I would study more and work harder than any other person in a given field, so all I needed was the perfect product or service that I believed in to sell. Purified mineral water was a great product. Although most people drank water straight out of their garden hoses back then, I saw the trend toward a healthier lifestyle shifting quickly.

But since I had set the appointment, and I was raised not to waste anyone's valuable time, I was not going to blow off the health club. I had heard from people that time is gold. In my experience, though, I've learned time is only worth the value you put on it. If you treat your time as gold, you will value it as much as gold. If you treat time as platinum, you will value it as much as platinum, and hopefully others will value it as platinum too. But if you waste time, time will lose all of its value. I've witnessed so many people wasting time, as if they had all of the time in the world. Time is irreplaceable, and if you have the slightest desire to become successful on any plane in life, you damn well better learn to place value on it.

My father was one of my earliest teachers who drilled the concept of time being valuable into me at a very early age. My dad was never late for anything. We were not socially active as a family, but if there was an appointment, we'd be there early. I remember one year when I was working at a restaurant washing dishes at about the age of fourteen, a blinding snowstorm came in over our town. I heard my father yelling, "Let's go. It's time to leave for work. You'll be late."

I said, "Dad, the restaurant won't open today."

He said, "Well, if it does open, you'll be there for work. Now get your butt in the car." We drove approximately fifteen miles to the restaurant and didn't see a single car on the road. The owner stuck her head out the partially opened door and said they had been stuck there all night because the snow was too bad to drive home. I looked back at my dad's car and asked the owner to please tell him the restaurant would not be open today and that I was not needed; otherwise, he might leave me out there in the snow.

Time management is the most rudimentary skill you must master in life and in business. Time is precious, and if you value your time, you must learn how to manage it. You must get in the habit of making a list of everything that needs to be done on the following day and allocate a specific amount of time to invest in each task. Prioritize the things that are most important, and have a time or date allocated for completion. Every morning you must make time to review your daily schedule before starting your day. I always plan the following day the night before, setting time-allotments for each meeting, event, activity, and so on, which is also how I scheduled my job interviews. I gave myself a generous allowance for others' tardiness and took a book to interviews, just in case.

I have read a ton of biographies and books on success, self-help, self-improvement, and every other subject that is related to self-development. I have always had an appetite for knowledge that never will be satisfied. As soon as I finish one book, I buy another. In my youth, I'd try to save them and read them over and over until I felt I could lecture on the material. I tried even the craziest of ideas in the real world to analyze their validity. I kept the things that worked and fit my personality, values, and style, and the rest I filed away. When I became more successful, and the cost of a book wasn't an issue any longer, I would leave the book wherever I finished it, so someone else could reap the same benefits as I did. So, needless to say (but I'll say it anyway), I have read numerous books on time management.

Time management is much simpler than most people imagine. The challenge for most people is being accountable for their time. A lot of people want to do things by the seat of their pants, and they don't want to be in a committed time frame. There are 168 hours in a week, and if you learn to effectively manage your time, you will be able to achieve all your goals.

Knowing how to manage your time is a necessity for your entire life; it's not just important for business. You should schedule time for every part of your life—pleasure, leisure, family, spouse, kids, and so on. If you do this, you will guarantee yourself quality time with all the people who are important to you. I schedule everything into my day, and I am absolutely sure I am going to accomplish whatever my objective is during that time. So, it goes without saying I would never have flaked out on my second job interview with the health club that day.

When I walked through the front door of the health club, I thought I had just entered the pearly gates of heaven! I immediately knew I was my father's son (my father was a world-class womanizer, which was the cause of my parents' divorce); there were girls, girls, and more girls, all wearing tight sexy outfits, looking fit and healthy while working out to great music. What's more, I was one of only two men in the joint. Thank you, Lord; thank you, thank you, I thought, looking up at the ceiling. This was unlike any health club I had ever been in. No sweaty grunting, cursing, or smelly men here. This work-out area was filled with princesses with big hair and fluorescent leotards.

Later, I was informed I was lucky to be interviewing on a women-only day because back then, some health clubs allowed only one gender in on any given day. In this club, men's days were on Tuesdays, Thursdays, Saturdays, and every other Sunday. Women's days were Mondays, Wednesdays, Fridays, and every other Sunday. There was a small work-out area on the other side of the lobby for those who wanted to work out on the days not assigned to them, but the equipment and access were limited. The company had several locations with different women's and men's schedules to accommodate members' schedules as well.

I was sold on the health-club industry immediately, and all thoughts of selling water drained completely out of my mind. The image of my mother's smiling face was replaced by what looked like a delirious reimagining of a hair-metal video—all perms, headbands, free weights, leg warmers, and neon exercise outfits. They wouldn't need to sell me on the job; I was already thinking of ways I could sell them on hiring me. This was nothing like the old sweaty gyms I had come to associate with the industry. In fact, it had never occurred to me that a health club could be a place with so many beautiful, sexy, health-and-fitness-conscious women. Sign me up now!

During the interview, I learned the salary was a draw against future sales, and if I didn't sell, I would go broke and quickly lose the job. At that point, I didn't care. I would have paid them every penny I had to let me work there. I was also informed I would be working in the club only three-and-a-half days a week, but I would be there from morning to close to get my forty hours in. I don't remember much of anything else that transpired in the interview, other than the interviewer was so excited, he ran upstairs to get his boss to interview me as well. They offered me the job and asked whether I could start immediately. I wasn't weighing my options then, and I certainly wasn't considering what would be best for my future. I just wanted to start as soon as possible and stay in the health-club business forever.

But when I came back down to earth, I had to make a decision. Either I was going to sell water-purifying systems door to door, or I was going to spend my twelve-hour days surrounded by sexy women in skintight leotards, listening to rock 'n' roll. Even though it was the disco era, the club I worked in played rock 'n' roll, unless there was an aerobics class. This was before music became a big issue in health clubs, from members wanting to have a say about what was piped through the loudspeakers, to artists and record companies demanding royalties.

I would love to be able to say I agonized over the decision all night, but that would be a lie. It was easy for me to forget my mother's advice and common sense when she was hundreds of miles away. At the age of nineteen, most single men have only two thoughts in their heads—sex and food. As long as this job could pay me enough to eat, I was in. So, I entered the business enthusiastically, never thinking it was the start of a long and lucrative career that would span more than thirty-five years.

I showed up for my first day ready to start my new life. Unfortunately, I must have missed the part of the interview when

I was told I would actually be working on men's days and not women's. Although I was temporarily devastated, my spirits were quickly lifted again by my trainer, who divulged some of the perks of the health-club business—one being that the small work-out side would be packed with ladies on men's days, and another being that some of my coworkers, including the aerobics instructors and receptionists, would be female. The sun began to shine once again. The last thing I wanted to do for twelve to sixteen hours a day was look at guys working out.

The first couple of months were nothing short of awesome. I met a ton of great people and learned the ins and outs of health and fitness as well as the health-club business. I realized most of the things I thought I knew about lifting weights were wrong. For the first time in my life, I had to start thinking about my eating habits. My folks were both from the rural South and brought their bad habits with them to Chicago (where I was born and lived until the age of eleven), so we were raised on southern comfort food from birth. Biscuits and gravy, fried chicken, barbeque ribs, and coleslaw were staples at our table—no green salads or smoothies for us. My mother fed us food that would stick to our ribs, as well as our arteries. Even my football coaches just said, "Get big, eat boy, and get big," when it came to dietary advice. They didn't know about proteins, carbohydrates, or good fats. All we knew was beans with fatback or ham hocks and cornbread, and the bigger the bowl, the better.

I was spending all of my free time chasing ladies and studying the business. It turned out I had an insatiable appetite for women, just like my father. I was living the life of a rock star, and it wasn't costing me a dime—most of my dates happened in the club itself (and that was a good thing because I was still broke). I was extremely lucky, even when it came to dating, because all the guys I worked with loved tall blondes with big boobs, and I loved short brunettes with great butts.

We were called counselors back then, and as a counselor, I could visit the other clubs, which meant I could visit clubs with an opposite schedule as mine. I was young, good looking, and in a candy store full of sexy women, so when I was not in a workshop or seminar, and it was my day off, I was health-club hopping.

I quickly found out how important sales were in the health-club business. I saw some of the sales guys driving Corvettes, Mustangs, Cadillacs, and other nice cars. They wore expensive clothes and flashy jewelry—you know, the usual bling associated with used-car salesmen. A light went on, and I started to realize that girls were not the only reason guys worked (although I still thought they were first on the list). I quickly realized that if I was going to make a good living in this industry, I would have to learn how to do what I was hired to do—sell memberships. I was having a great time and loving my newfound paradise, but I was also worried the owner would get wind of my escapades and give me the boot if I didn't start producing (selling) fast. I needed to prove I was a good sales-man and bring value to the company, and I needed to earn some real money to be able to afford a decent place to live.

Like all businesses, health clubs rely on sales to be successful. Nothing happens until a sale is made. Salaries, rents, leases, and mortgages all depend on sales. If you want guaranteed success in any industry, learn how to effectively sell your product or service. More sales will grow any business and bring it long-term security and prosperity. You can create the greatest product or service in the world, but if you fail to sell it in the marketplace, it will be des-tined for the great-ideas graveyard.

I was very fortunate this company had the foresight to hire a company to design a sales system for them. I have always been skeptical of really polished, fast-talking, slick people selling their snake oil and I wasn't about to sell anything like those kind of "salespeople." I learned quickly that people preferred a salesper-son who talked and thought as they did. Just being myself—a guy with very limited previous experience in sales—could work to my advantage. I passionately loved my product, eagerly wanted to help people, and loved learning. I found myself working for a company that provided an abundance of membership-sales training to any employee willing to put forth some effort. After only a few short months, I made a commitment to learn an ironclad system of selling that would complement my personality and represent my values.

The company had six locations around town. Since I didn't have a car, I hitchhiked to each location for a variety of membership-sales training courses. Every manager had a different style of teaching and a different style of selling, and like a sponge, I wanted to soak up every drop of information I could get my hands on. So on my days off, I visited each location for eye-opening lessons designed to make me a more successful salesman. To this day, I am grateful to the owner of that company, who recognized that a well-trained staff is happier and far more productive than a bunch of loose cannons.

I believe anyone can do anything he or she wants if he or she just knew the system, and my sales philosophy followed the same theory: anyone could sell any product as long as he or she knew the right sales system. Additionally, anyone with passion and a willingness to work hard could surely succeed. Working forty hours a week pays the bills, and that's great. But the time you put in after that will pave the road for your future. Learn to embrace your drive to succeed, and be prepared and willing to work longer hours, holidays and weekends, especially if you're not a parent yet. I guarantee you this golden nugget will serve you well.

As I started learning more about the health-club business, I gradually realized I was the most fortunate person on earth for getting started in the business in this particular health-club chain. I found a job I loved, and I knew it would mirror my lifestyle. I was going to be an evangelist for health and fitness, giving the gift of health and fitness to everyone, and along the way, I would make a modest but very comfortable living for myself and future family.

Win-win is a guiding principle you can apply to every arena of your life. If a scale is tipped too far to one side, there will be winners, and there will be losers. This scenario of winners and losers breeds resentment in the slighted party. Never make your employees, clients, or prospects feel as if they are on the losing side of a transaction. Both parties have to walk away feeling like winners, and your transactions will pay dividends for life. Over the years I have read several studies that explore this topic but one in particular comes to mind, two participants had to divide a large sum of money. The caveat was that one participant would choose how to split the money, that is, who received how much, and the other would decide whether both participants would keep the money or both would walk away with nothing. The facilitators of the study found if the first participant tried to take more than 70 percent, the second participant would decline the money, and neither participant would receive a penny. People just cannot stand to let someone take advantage of them, and they are willing to deny themselves a reward if they think it will teach the other party a lesson. I knew this job was going to be a huge win-win for all parties involved.

During my time as a sales trainee, sales counselors (a.k.a. salespeople) were able to monitor most sales presentations by placing a sign on the table stating, "This presentation may be monitored for quality customer service and training purposes," which is a practice still in place today for customer service and sales calls. Monitoring an ongoing sales interaction is a quick way to improve the effectiveness of a sales presentation and even helps modify sales training to accommodate what we had learned in previous sessions. The primary reason for the monitoring was to teach new sales counselors the tricks of the trade and have them ready to do a TO (take-over) if the counselor couldn't close the sale. A TO is used most frequently when a salesperson is having a hard time closing the sale but a colleague or manager can still salvage the deal by taking over the presentation. These days, the practice of monitoring presentations is hotly contested because some view it as unethical due to privacy issues, but its effectiveness makes it a fairly common tactic still used in most industries.

Sales training should be significantly more professional in 2017, but I want to make sure you have a complete picture of the evolution of professional sales. The profession of sales has evolved from a maniacal focus on closing the sale at all costs to listening to customers and showing them how a product or service can meet their needs. Unfortunately, for most counselors in those days, commissions were more important than ethical practices or relationship-building between the salesperson and the new member. Today, selling is a craft with deep ties to multiple disciplines. The average salesperson in the 1980s had no concept of the psychology of selling, which is a shorthand term I use to encompass a school of thought related to professionally selling products and services based on the needs and wants of consumers. If you don't believe in what you are selling, you will have a very difficult time convincing your prospects to believe in it. As a professional salesperson, you want to demonstrate the value of your product, and when you think of value, you have to think of more than just its momentary value—products and services have emotional value as well.

A sale takes place when one person transfers his or her enthusiasm about a product or service to another person. A professional salesperson or marketer knows people buy for emotional reasons and justify their purchases with logical reasons. Look at all beer commercials. Instead of showing you what a beer drinker actually looks like—fat bellies, with cirrhosis of the liver and a hangover—beer commercials show you the fantasy: beautiful women, exotic locations, and many friends. Do you really think people buy beer because they think it is good for them? Of course not; they buy into the promise of a good time. Consumers believe buying the beer will allow them to feel good, hang out with buddies, and have a shot at getting a sexy, hot lady to join them. But nobody would dream of admitting this. A consumer will tell you he or she bought the beer because it tastes good or was on sale.

From the manager's office, I would listen to the full spectrum of salespeople at work. I listened to them begin with an interview of the prospect, all the way through the end of the presentation, with their closing techniques. Some were as smooth as butter, and others were as rough as a rocky road, but I learned something from all of them. The lessons about what not to do were just as valuable as the ones that taught me what a flawless sales presentation sounded like. The company had a training program for their sales system, and most of the counselors stuck to it like glue. I could easily hear when the counselors would get tripped up and make costly mistakes because they couldn't improvise when things got off script. These guys failed to understand the system was just that: a system, not a canned speech.

When someone develops any kind of system, it is meant to be a guide. The architect has no way of accounting for every personality, question, concern, fear, emotion, and so on that can arise. This is where your personal development as a professional salesperson must come in and take over. For example, I have provided a rudimentary version of my sales system on my company's website, healthclubmarketingmmc.com, as a free download to draw visitors to our site. This mini sales system has the basic components of a professional sales presentation and can guide anyone through a professional membership-sales presentation. What it doesn't do is give you all of the nuances necessary to go from a novice to a professional; it is those nuances that separate the kids from the grown-ups, but the download provides the reader with an awesome foundation.

The free download teaches the reader to ask ten basic questions to overcome the four core objections: time, money, spouse, and I need to think about it. If you simply follow the steps outlined, even the worst salespeople on earth will close 20 percent of the guests they see. But if you want your closing percentage to go through the roof, you need to ask at least fifty quality questions. You need to know what to ask, where in the presentation to ask, when to probe deeper, when to start asking test-closing questions, and on and on, which I will teach you in chapter three of this book. The difference in the level of skill between an interviewer and a great interviewer is relative to the difference in level of skill between a general practitioner and a neurosurgeon. And never forget, everything is relative; not only is there an enormous difference in the level of skill involved, but there is also an enormous difference in compensation.

Offices (which were really closing stations) in the 1980s were sometimes set up to subtly intimidate the prospect. You still see an example of this in the way banks use grand lobbies, big desks, and gold details to elevate the importance of their salespeople. There were big desks in our club's offices with an executive chair behind each desk and two small chairs directly in front and across from the sales counselor. The idea was to give an authoritative look to the person behind the desk while diminishing the power of the prospect. I know this sounds funny today, but there was far less education readily available to the average consumer back then, especially concerning the psychology of selling. Another peculiar thing I noticed about the setup of the offices was the low-hanging light above the prospect's chair, as if he or she were in an interrogation room. Prospects would sit in small chairs, sweating under a hot bulb, looking up at the sales counselor, appearing all powerful, behind a big desk in a comfortable chair, with an air-conditioning vent at his or her back.

The strategies for selling to people in the 1980s were wildly different from what they are in 2017. Some of those tactics of the 1980s would not work today, but others work even better today, because consumers have been conditioned to them. Instead of relying on outdated gimmicks, a well-trained professional salesperson will mirror the prospect, and not separate him or herself from the prospect. Remember people tend to relate to and trust people who are same as them. The last thing you want is something in between you and the prospect.

There used to be a saying in the industry back in the 1980s: "They will leave either signing or crying." Today, I look back at some of the things we considered tricks of the trade, and I have to laugh, although a lot of those techniques worked really well, like how people were so programmed to bend to the will of the authoritarian behind the desk. It is learning a ton of little details like how consumers react in certain situations that will catapult your career into the atmosphere. Don't focus on all the things you need to learn; focus on the experience of learning. By the time you finish this book you will be far better prepared than the majority of your coworkers and competitors. I will give you the tools you need to be successful, and since you bought, and are reading this book, you are obviously willing to put the work in, which in my humble opinion is the winning combination for success, that is, education and hard work.

I have learned through the years that the 80/20 rule (Pareto principle) applies to many situations you will face. Eighty percent of people will not apply themselves completely, and 20 percent will; this is why 80 percent of the wealth is owned by 20 percent of the population. I am happy to say that most of the things I learned back then in my health-club days were very valuable to my career. They turned out to be important components in the overall picture of my success. Through the years of endless study and research, I have taken bits and pieces of knowledge from numerous great sources and compiled them into what I consider to be the very best way to market and sell any health-and-fitness product and service in today's marketplace, while maintaining the dignity and integrity of a brand, a business, and the prospect.

You won't sell to everyone, but you will sell to most people if you learn a great system. If you get to where you sell eight out of every ten prospects (i.e., only fail to lock up the relationship 20 percent of the time), you will be wealthier than you ever dreamed. So learn your craft, put the time in. I don't waste my time on theories and principles that don't work in the real world, so all you'll learn in this book will be those tools that are applicable in the real world.

In the first few years of my career, I vigorously pursued my passions (women and knowledge). I was becoming one of the top three salespeople every month within our company because of how eager I was to learn soaking up knowledge at work and during my days off. Unfortunately, I was also becoming infamous for my after-hours indulgences, like the time the owner's daughter came in for an early-morning workout only to find me passed out completely naked on the lobby's couch after a late-night pool party in the club. Late at night, my common sense would fly out the window, and more than once, I was caught doing things that would have resulted in my being fired had I not been a consistently good (and getting better every day) salesman. Although I was not the only employee guilty of this in the 1980s, I was surely the most frequent. I can't help it; I love women, and I was enjoying my youth.

I will share with you an embarrassing time to highlight how important being a top producer was, and the crap I got away with, because I was making the company so much money. We had a pump room that housed all of the motors, pumps and supplies for the wet area, that is, swimming pool, Jacuzzi, steam room, sauna and eucalyptus room that was located around the back of the spa. A lot of the employees used it as a make-out room. One day I was down there with an aerobics instructor. She was on her knees in front of me, and my head was laid back in sheer ecstasy, when bam! The door flew open, and standing there staring straight at us was one of the VPs and about three other guys. Talk about your awkward situation. I quickly maneuvered my friend around me to shelter her face and went back upstairs fully expecting to be fired. A day, week, and then a month went by, and I never heard a word. Later I heard those guys with the VP were looking to buy into the company. Whoops! But that was the spa business in the 1980s— one wild time.

But hindsight proved reluctant acceptance of my behavior was the opposite of what I should have been striving for. My sales numbers were getting better and better. I was grossing more than the other two or three sales counselors combined, but I still wasn't getting promoted. With the proper training, any muscle can grow in size and strength; my sales muscles were getting stronger, but my overall compensation and commission structure was still the same as when I had first started. I wanted a bigger piece of the pie. I wanted some guys to train myself so I could get a percentage of their sales (a.k.a. override). I wanted the extra income from sales I had an indirect hand in. I had been training my coworkers and closing a lot of their sales in TOs, but I wasn't getting compensated for it. At first, I didn't mind at all, but when I saw people who had far inferior sales skills to mine and who worked far fewer hours than I did being promoted into management, I started getting frustrated.

I asked my manager for a promotion weekly with the determination of a still-young kid, and every week, I received the same answer: "Not now. We're not currently promoting managers at this location. Besides, so-and-so has been with us far longer than you; we can't promote you over him. We'll throw your name in the hat and see what happens at the next executive meeting." It was all total BS meant to distract me from the fact that I wasn't getting into management because of my after-hours shenanigans. My arrogance wasn't helping either. I truly believed my sales prowess alone should guarantee me a position in management. One thing you'll learn in business is that sales are king, and you will be able to get away with a lot if you are producing, but not every great salesperson is management material. There is a reason why universities have entire programs in business management. Managing a business along with its staff takes a skill set that must be learned.

The management team of the company must have been laughing at me behind closed doors at their weekly meetings. What I didn't understand at the time was my actions were speaking much louder than my words. In their eyes, I was the furthest thing from management material that had ever walked through the club's doors. I was simply some reckless party boy who was being tolerated only because he made the club a ton of money. But I would never be promoted. And you know what? They were right. I was an earner, but I was masking my passion for the job with alcohol and liaisons with my coworkers and the club's members. My partying ways were distracting my superiors' focus from the fire that burned inside of me and yearned for success above everything else. I had what it took to be successful in the business, but I hadn't yet learned how to show my potential to others—all they could see was the wild side of me. I'm sure they were more concerned with the money I might have cost them by being in a management position than the potential earnings I could have generated leading a team. And even worse, what kind of an example would I have been as a team leader?

Early in my career, I benefited from creative, outside-the-box thinking. I knew the only way to achieve my version of success was to either become a manager or sell more memberships—in other words, bring more value to more people. I brought real value to this business, which I could have quantified and used to my advantage. If I had stopped to think for a minute about what it was I really wanted, I could have realized my true goal of increasing my income by speaking with the owner (who had an open-door policy long before it was the trendy thing to do) and negotiated a higher commission based on my impressive sales numbers. I could have achieved my goal without having to spend weeks and weeks campaigning for a job I was not ready for at the time and still increased my earnings: win-win. Unfortunately (or maybe fortunately), I wasn't privy to this technique at that stage in my life.

I thought there was a set path to success: salesperson, assistant manager, manager, director of sales, vice president, and owner. Ignorantly, I thought everyone received the same commission structure, which was inked into an unalterable contract that would limit my income until I received a promotion to assistant manager. But I should have been asking myself the question all great businesspeople learn to ask: How can I get what I want while giving the other person what he or she wants? Every human being is always asking ourselves questions, but sometimes, we fail to ask ourselves the correct questions. We must learn to ask ourselves better questions. Had I asked myself better questions and then asked upper management better questions, I may have secured the position I desperately sought. The bottom line is if you bring value to the negotiating table, you can certainly come away a winner. Just prepare your presentation beforehand, and know exactly what it is you want. Compensation can come in many forms. Don't just think in monetary terms; think of perks as another option.

I worked at that health club for about a year, managed to consistently maintain the title as a top producer, and took advantage of all the training that was available. As I have said, I love learning. I had been selling memberships for a while at that point, and I had learned a lot. But my education was getting stagnant. I was thirsty to learn, but I had already drunk all the juice that company offered. I needed to learn more, and I wanted to learn business management. I was going to have to take a break from the club business and attend an institution of higher learning for the academic skills I lacked. So, I took a year off and went back to school.

I enrolled in a community college and only took classes that directly pertained to my goals. By that time, I viewed a college education differently. Before, I had thought of a college education as a necessity to get a good job and achieve my goals, whereas now, I viewed a college education as a tool to help me build a foundation. No longer was I interested in spending four years of my life studying subjects unrelated to real-world scenarios. I would pursue my passions of women and wealth in the health-and-fitness industry; I just needed to acquire some tools to help me do the job far better than anyone else.

So, I spoke with management and informed them I would be leaving for a while, and I went on a one-year total immersion in the academic side of business with the conviction I would surface with the tools necessary to successfully manage any health club on earth. During that entire year, all I focused on were my studies and getting back into the club. I felt at home, at peace, and as if I belonged when I was in the club. The club was my territory, and like a lion missing his pride, I was missing the health-club lifestyle I was born for. After one year, almost to the day, I went straight back to the club and got my old job back. Of course, I was armed with a strategy this time. I would work for a few months as a counselor to get my sales chops back, and then, I would address upper management about a managerial position once again.

All was fantastic; I started selling as if I had never been gone. I was far better than I had been in the past at lead generation and was coming up with a ton of different ways to prospect on my own to bring guests in the door without costing the club a dime. I wore my uniform everywhere and talked up the club and health and fitness to every person who would listen. The sales clerk in the mall, the waitress in the food court, the pizza-delivery man—if someone had a job and spoke to me, he or she left with an appointment for a free workout at the club. I was rockin'. No one was even close to me in numbers of sales. There was only one snag. I still was my father's son, and since the club was now coed, it was very difficult for me not to entertain my second passion—women.

A few months after I returned, the owner decided to put a suspended aerobics floor over the main work-out area. He really understood trends and knew he had to get a better aerobics program if he wanted to stay competitive in the marketplace. What a fantastic idea, I thought. Now there were even more beautiful ladies in the clubs because all of the aerobics instructors rotated throughout the six clubs. I'll tell you: my life just kept getting better and better.

We counselors were sent to other clubs to work while our location was closed for the renovation. I was sent to a club managed by a relative of one of the vice presidents, and this manager and I just didn't get along. Part of my reputation included speaking my mind and not being afraid to knuckle up. On a couple of occasions, I had gotten into fistfights over the short time I worked for the club so to say the least; the first time we disagreed, he was extremely worried and called the VP of operations (his brother-in-law). I immediately received a call, and the VP said, "Chuck, do me a favor, and go back to the club, and watch over things for us. We will still pay you, and all you have to do is hang out." What he was really saying was, "Chuck, go hang out at the other club, and don't kill my relative." I loved the idea and said it was not a problem.

The company was still paying my draw, but it was nothing without the commissions and bonuses, so I started presenting to everyone who came into the club. When past members stopped by to see what was going on, I sold them memberships. When current members stopped by to see whether we were open yet, I sold them extensions to their existing memberships. Plumbers, electricians, phone-repair guys, inspectors, subcontractors, tile people, carpet guys, welders—I sold them all memberships. If you came anywhere near that club, you were buying a membership. And better yet, no one ever complained that I was harassing them, because they all felt my sincerity and concern for their health and fitness. The executives were flabbergasted. I sold more memberships during construction, while the club was closed, than some of the other clubs in the chain did, including the one I had just left, which were fully operational and fully staffed.

After construction was completed, and we were officially back up and selling, I wanted to readdress the subject of my getting into management. To my dismay, when I presented the owner with my management request, I was denied yet again. I still didn't fully understand the magnitude of negative self-promotion I was giving myself as a playboy and a bit of a hothead. I knew everyone else was partaking in extracurricular activities, and they were in management, so what was the big deal about me? I just didn't see it. At the time, I egotistically thought maybe the upper management saw me as a threat because I was moving fast, but I thought I had already proven myself. Unfortunately, my actions were speaking louder than my numbers.

My ego just couldn't handle it, so I resigned. I hated to leave because I really loved everyone in the company, and I had learned so much, but I was twenty-two and a forward thinker, so I needed forward movement. My reputation as a salesperson was well known to all of our competitors because no one shopping our club ever made it to my competitors for a second appointment. I closed prospects on their first visit to my club because I knew I might not get a second chance, and my competitor had just let the sale go. I used to say, "Be backs aren't greenbacks." A prospect is most susceptible to your presentation when he or she first comes into your club or business. He or she is more emotionally involved and connected with your product on the first visit than at any other time. You must grab the opportunity to get him or her engaged with your product or service. There is no tomorrow when it comes to sales.

When I started to put feelers out for another health club that could use my services, I realized both sides of my reputation preceded me. Everyone knew I was a fantastic salesperson, but they also knew I lived outside the box. All the clubs knew if I came to work for them, I was going to be a handful. It would be a challenge to tame or at a minimum contain this wild stallion. On the other hand, if the club took a chance on me, the potential for growth was beyond anyone's imagination. Most were apprehensive, to say the least, but all of them really wanted to give it a try.

The first place I thought I would try was a club in a strip mall not far from my apartment. I knew the chain of clubs and was also aware they were part of a national company as opposed to locally owned, which meant more chances of upward mobility for me. It was a smaller club than I was used to. My last club had a huge wet area, including an indoor swimming pool. This club was all on one level and had a smaller version of almost everything, other than a wet area. When I walked in, I just blew past the front desk and went straight for the offices to look for the manager. On my way, I saw an old friend who taught *tae kwon do* at a school where I had studied in Knoxville. We talked for a few minutes, and then the manager came up to us, shook my hand, and introduced himself.

He said, "Hey, Chuck, are you here to shop us?" Shopping your competitor is when you go to another business similar to your own and take a tour to see the facilities and compare pricing and pre-sentations. This is something all businesses and their sales staff *must do.* You must know your competition to know your own place in the market. If you are in charge of marketing, you will call this a competitive overview. I had shopped this particular health club several months before. I responded to the manager's question, wanting to get straight to the point, "No, I'm looking for a career move into a management position."

It turned out that getting a management position was as easy as walking through the door. I was lucky because the current assistant manager was not pulling his weight, and his head was already on the chopping block and just like that, I was the new assistant manager. Finally, I would be able to get my hands on a bigger piece of the pie. But the job came with a warning not to let my bachelor lifestyle interfere with the sales. This manager knew he would make ten times as much money with me as a partner than he would with any other salesperson as an assistant. I would only bolster his position at the club and continue my climb up the corporate ladder, right behind him. I am not the kind of guy to take my friend's job; I am way too loyal for that, but I made it well known I wanted upward momentum. I had no problem pushing him up the ladder ahead of me as long as he didn't try to keep me down.

We got along great, and I have to say my position as assistant manager did not interfere with my responsibilities to my libido. We had some unbelievable parties in that club. In my first club, we had a lot of movie stars, professional wrestlers, and musicians working out, and a ton of celebrities stopping in for workouts while they were in Nashville for some session, movie, or event because the club was located in Greenhills, an upscale neighborhood with high-end shopping and restaurants. Greenhills is next to Brentwood, where a lot of country-music stars lived in the 1980s, so it was a hopping place to work, live, or visit. This new club, however, was in a middle-class neighborhood and had a lot of blue-collar members. But I fit in anywhere because it was all about women, fitness, and money to me, and as long as those three components were involved, I was happy. And for a while, I *was* happy.

Something was missing though, this health-club chain did not offer the same kinds of educational courses as the previous one had, and I felt my knowledge of membership sales would soon flat line in an industry that was being reinvented with each passing day. As much as I liked having fun, I love learning more. I didn't feel I was growing or learning anything. I was studying on my own—reading books and listening to tapes—but I wasn't getting hands-on training. The guys at the club were great, but they were still using techniques I had learned in the beginning as canned presentations. I knew sooner or later, I would resign, even though

I previously would have done anything for a management position. I guess I was really learning what my true priorities were.

I decided it was time to strike out on my own as a consultant and try my hand at working with a few of the little independent clubs in town. This career change felt as if it would satisfy my emotional need for growth. I knew enough about the health-club business, having been a top-grossing salesman for about three years in a competitive market. I could easily sell owners on the idea of hiring me, or at least giving me a chance to prove myself over the course of a few weeks. I was willing to work for free for one week to prove myself. I had already been learning about risk reversal and investments with no downside. I knew there were very few true no-risk opportunities for businesspeople, so I was determined to make my services absolutely risk-free. If I did not produce in a week, they wouldn't owe me a dime. Thirty-five years later I still work the same way.

Nearly every investment a person makes has a potential downside. There is a school of thought you must take enormous risk to get huge returns on your investments; this is more of a myth than a reality. You do need to be smart and educate yourself, but there are numerous ways to receive enormous returns on your investments if you get out of your own way and start thinking outside the box. As an owner, look for people and companies to do business with who offer the least downside and the most potential upside. The key to success for the individual or company is to make your product or service risk-free to your customers, which is why I present my services with absolutely no downside to the club owner.

I had also been studying the importance of research. So before I left my job, I researched every club in town. I found several mom-and-pop health clubs and knew my best shot would be with one of these clubs. I started calling around and set some appointments with the owners. I didn't have a media kit back then, but I knew if anyone sat down with me for twenty minutes, I would blow him or her away with my knowledge of membership sales. I had taken what I had learned up to that point and started developing a professional sales system. People thought they knew me because of stories they had heard, but no one really knew who I was or what I was about. I think most people were attracted to me because I was so ambitious, honest, and my enthusiasm was contagious. I was far more than a daydreamer; I worked every day on my craft. I studied and implemented what I was learning to see whether it held up in the real world. I kept what worked universally and discarded the rest.

A couple of days after my resignation, I was consulting with a small gym (not a full service health club, like the ones I had been working for before) owned and operated by a deeply religious family. The club was very small and was located in the basement of an office building downtown. To say the business was slow would be far too generous. This business was dead. It was a dark, dull dungeon that needed life badly. Health clubs need members; they need energy; and most of all, they need light. Psychology plays an enormous role in business, and you must know a little about the effects every aspect of your business has on the psyches of your members and guests. People who struggle with weight may also struggle with bouts of depression. The last thing overweight people want to do is work out in a morgue, so I made an agreement with the owner that the revenue from my first few sales would go straight into the rejuvenation of the club. The most important thing was to repaint the place and try to brighten everything up.

I put together a corporate membership for all of the downtown businesses and went door to door. Within a month or so, the club started getting some life. During the day, the club was holding its own, but there was no evening crowd. I desperately tried to build up the evening traffic, but it was like pulling teeth. By that time, I was learning the power of questions and the importance of gathering data. So, I put together a questionnaire for my members and offered to give everyone who participated a free week-long pass to the gym to give to anyone he or she wanted. This was a win-win because the member got to do something nice for someone he or she knew; the owner got a guest who could be converted into a member; the guest got a free week to work out; and I got my data.

From the interviews, I learned an invaluable lesson about location. Most people wanted to leave downtown as soon as the clock struck five, and they didn't want to return downtown until the next morning, which meant we would be able to build a great lunch crowd and grow the morning crowd, but the industry's normal rush hours of 4:00 p.m. to 8:00 p.m. were going to be nonexistent for the most part. A lot of metropolitan city officials struggle with keeping people downtown after 5:00 p.m., but changing perceptions of city-living doesn't happen overnight. Today, most cities are developing their city-living and are doing their best to keep people downtown, but I didn't have time to start a trend of downtown-living; I needed action, excitement, and variety now.

I really liked the owner, and I had made a huge impact on his business, but I wasn't happy. The pay was great, and the owners really showed their appreciation, but I felt my hands were tied with this project, and since it wasn't my club, I wasn't about to spend the next twenty years in the trenches just to pay the bills. Besides, I didn't have the comforts and liberties that may have made the job more attractive to me. My work took place behind the scenes, and the perks were few and far between—not to mention my client was a devout Christian who would have seen my lifestyle as, shall I say, sinful and not conducive to his beliefs. Again, I felt myself going stir-crazy because even though I could see growth in my new career path—the field of consulting—I still felt something was missing. Did I really want to go in the trenches time and time again, busting my butt and working sixteen-hour days, for a few thousand dollars a month? If this was my dream, why did I feel so empty and unfulfilled?

As always, though, I did learn a lot and grew in the couple of short months I worked there as a consultant. A local newspaper did a piece on health clubs and their growing popularity, quoting my knowledge on membership sales and presenting me as a local expert in the health-club industry, which was a huge arrow in my quiver for future work and a fantastic line for my ever-expanding résumé. This was the first time my ideas about asking ten basic questions to overcome the four core objections (time, money, spouse, and the "I need to think about it" excuse for not joining today) were published. By far, this is the easiest sales system to lock up relationships with new members because you know prospects' objections before the prospects even know they are going to say them. This article was published around 1985.

I knew now I wanted to focus on high-end health clubs in residential neighborhoods, where I would have access to larger numbers of potential customers. There was one other big chain of health clubs in town, so I knocked on their door, and to no one's surprise, they eagerly entertained the prospect of my joining their team. This time, I was prepared to stand my ground and pursue only a general manager's position. I knew my own value at that point and had a track record of three for three success stories to share. I was told they would hire me as a manager, but first, I had to go through a thirty-day training program in Nashville with one of the owners and then transfer to Kentucky and undergo a three-month training program with one of their best managers in their flagship club.

This particular chain of health clubs fit me like a glove. The clubs were big and beautiful, with all of the amenities, including racquetball. The owners were just like me at the time: they were obsessed with success, growth, and variety. Another bonus was that their lifestyles mirrored mine, so no one would worry about what I did in my free time. The owners were the biggest womanizers I'd ever seen. Hell, they made me look like a saint—OK, a saint might be pushing it. But in all seriousness, this group knew the business, which gave me confidence that I was about to get an advanced education on a whole different level. To put it mildly, I was excited to enter this new chapter of my career!

CHAPTER 2

THE FITNESS EXPLOSION

I started at the new club immediately; I have never been one to let grass grow under my feet. This club was about twenty miles away from the first health club where I worked in Nashville. Almost all the seasoned staff knew me before I even stepped in the club, which made the transition easier since I didn't have to prove myself. The club was awesome; it was huge, and these owners were ahead of the curve when it came to club layout, style, and décor, and they were more up to date on the trends of the industry. The location was also great because it was not far from a major highway. There was ample parking, and the staff was hot: these were all key components for a successful health club.

The only thing I could see missing in this mammoth building was members. What a shame—this enormous, gorgeous club with state-of-the-art equipment and amenities was dead. These owners really knew how to make it presentable but had failed to learn the most important aspect of a successful business—having a finely tuned sales system being used by a finely tuned sales team. They had the great-looking employees, but the employees lacked the necessary sales skills to put members in the club. This was the classic *Field of Dreams* nightmare. They had built it, but no one was coming. Now, it was crystal clear why the owners jumped on the idea of my coming onboard. They knew not only would I sell a ton of memberships, but I would share the sales system I had been developing with the entire company.

The health club I loved was a little behind in some things, but it was far ahead in the things that mattered most—sales, service, and sanitation; what I would later coin as the three *S*'s of any brick-and-mortar business. Sales always come first because if you do not have members, then you don't have anyone to offer service to, nor do you have the revenue to hire someone to keep the place clean. Sales are the foundation of any business, but most owners are unaware of the successful systems available that can make the difference between thriving and barely surviving. Fortunately, the owners of this club knew their weakness and had taken the first step in rectifying it by hiring me.

This group had a forward-thinking approach, going on the offensive and solving the problem of the old racquetball-court clubs before anyone realized the problem existed. Declining attendance after the heyday of the 1970s left these racquetball clubs on the verge of bankruptcy, which not only would have resulted in the loss of the business but could have snowballed into the loss of the real estate. My new bosses would come in as partners with the original owners of the racquetball clubs for pennies on the dollar, tear out most of the courts, and put in the equipment and facilities necessary to convert the hollowed-out space into proper health clubs geared to serve the new consumer, the fitness crowd, which was a very smart business decision.

The owners of this new club brokered the partnership between themselves and the racquetball-club owners on future revenue to cover their investment and leased the equipment, which made it an almost no-money-down investment; in short, they were able to see the direction of a trend, get out in front of it, and make a killing. Instead of waiting for a business to tank and buying up the space to rebuild a new club, all they had to do was rebrand the old business and make sure to retain the customers who were still loyal to the racquetball club. The investment was minimal, but the returns were astronomical. Remember it is more profitable to get out in front of a trend than to start a trend. A lot of people want to create trends, and my hat goes off to them, but I have always focused on determining which way a new trend is going and getting out in front of it; that's where the money is.

The month in Nashville flew by, and in no time, the club was rockin'. The owners knew how to party and take care of their employees. That is another thing I can say about the first Nashville club where I started my career: they had parties at least every quarter, and their parties were epic. We had great food, open bars, dancing, and lots of hot beautiful girls. Between the six clubs, there were probably a couple hundred employees, and a lot of the girls brought friends. We were all young and wild; most people in the club business in the 1980s were party animals. You would think the opposite since we were all health conscious, but when Thursday nights came around (ladies' nights at most nightclubs), you could see half of our staff as well as half of our members in the nightclubs, partying their asses off. I learned very early on in my career that knowing the lifestyle patterns of our members would serve me well in how I recruited new members in the future.

These club owners at this new club threw a ton of money into advertisement, but the sales staff didn't have the sales acumen to lock up the relationships (close the sales). I, on the other hand, was a closing machine. People use to refer to me as the Hammer when it came to closing the sale; when no one else could close the sale, the manager brought me in to lock up the relationship. I wasn't referred to as the Hammer because I was loud, obnoxious, or forceful; it was because I was the guy to get the job done. I was constantly updating my sales system, just as an accountant adds to a ledger. I also removed techniques from my system if I found they didn't live up to their hype. I was determined to build a foolproof, professional way of locking up relationships. Let's face it: the staff you want representing your club should be attractive, fit, and energetic people who can sell. The challenge, as anyone in charge of hiring can attest is, you don't always get the cream-of-the-crop applicants who look great, have the drive necessary to succeed, and are willing to devote the time to learn a professional sales system on their own.

Management was where I wanted to be, not because I wanted to sit on my butt all day but so I could build a team of salespeople under me to leverage my time and quadruple my income as well as the income for my employers. I learned at a very young age that I must bring value to my employer, and the more value I brought, the more I would earn. Later, I took it one step further: if I brought more value to more people, I could earn even more. So, my focus was on bringing more value to my employer as well as to more people. I wanted to be in management because I knew I could accomplish both goals from a leadership position.

During that first month, I hustled my butt off, closing sales, doing TOs, and training the sales staff. I wanted this place to rock. It was beautiful, and people needed to enjoy it. I knew I was getting into management—whether I did anything here at the Nashville club or not—because that was in my contract, but I never needed a written contract to do my best. I know only one way in life, and that's to give 100 percent. A winner is always a winner; it doesn't take outside stimuli to get winners to excel because winners only knew acceleration. I wasn't getting bonuses or overrides on the staff I was training since technically, I was a trainee as well, but I was getting a whole lot more in return for my time than money. I was growing because these people needed, and were extremely grateful for the knowledge I shared with them.

It is important to always know what you really want out of any negotiation and believe it or not, even a job interview can be a negotiation. Do you want a guaranteed salary and if so, how much? Do you want an entry-level job that will possibly grow into a position in management, upper management, ownership, and so on? For example, money isn't always what you want or even what you need out of every negotiation. Sometimes, it can be perks like a coveted parking space, a flexible work schedule, or other intangibles that make the negotiation a win-win. Always think outside the box and know what you really want.

The clubs in Kentucky really needed help because they had just been recently acquired, and the owners had dumped a ton of borrowed money into the renovations. The plan was for me to move to Kentucky for an additional three-month training period under a manager in the flagship club. The club I trained in was managed by a man who masked his laziness by becoming everyone's good friend. He told everyone exactly what they wanted to hear and had absolutely no backbone whatsoever. Hiring butt-kissers like this kills your business, but owners hire them because they like them, and since some brownnosers are so well liked, they are rarely canned. Friendliness and likeability are two important components of sales, but they must be paired with knowledge and hard work. This guy lacked the latter two components, and once I spent a day with him observing his work ethic, I didn't like him at all. I have never been able to stomach liars or lazy people, and this guy was both.

Within a week, I was running circles around him using the skills I had been honing from the very first few weeks of my career. After he left everyday early in the evening to go to his apartment and relax after a long day of doing nothing, I was still hustling late into the night. Most health clubs are busiest between four o'clock and eight o'clock in the evening; no manager should ever leave a club before 9:00 p.m., unless he or she just doesn't care about the business. The most basic rules of owning or managing a business are to always be the first to arrive, the last to leave, and always pay yourself last. Later, I realized the only reason he had his job was because one of the owners (who knew the manager was baggage) was banging the manager's girlfriend, and the owner always knew where the manager was when he wanted to see the guy's girlfriend.

After my initial training which lasted maybe five or six weeks (far short of what was scheduled), I was called into the local owner's office and assigned the club I would be managing and, more importantly, be responsible for growing. At the time, I was completely unaware that I was being sent to the worst part of town, in the middle of an industrial park. I knew the express lane I was driving in was going to have a few potholes, but I didn't know the owners would task me with turning around a health club where the odds were completely stacked against me. I had already learned my lesson about the importance of location with the downtown gym. I was now about to learn about the numbers behind a health club's draw area (reachable market) and how they affect the bottom line. People don't drive more than five miles (within most city limits) to a health club to work out. Usually it's less, and occasionally more if the town is rural. But a five-mile radius is the perfect starting point for demographic studies. Basically, if the residential population is too small or if it is too transient for whatever reason, most marketing efforts are dramatically diminished. And when your most effective marketing tools can't do the trick, you're in trouble and going nowhere fast, unless you are innovative and always thinking outside the box. The company's marketing was run by the home office, but I knew immediately it was definitely failing here.

One of my biggest challenges was the location. The second was a lack of interest in the product as a whole due to the demographic makeup of the area. Back in the early to mid-1980s, fewer people were as health-and-fitness-conscious as they are today. Convincing a blue-collar worker who had just put in a nine-hour day of hard physical labor to come in and work out for an hour was like asking him or her to work an extra hour with no overtime pay. In the laborer's mind, his or her daily requirement for strength training was easily met five days of the week. Since this club was in an industrial park, blue-collar workers were the customers I had to recruit as members. I thought back to the early days in Nashville, when I had sold memberships to farmers in overalls, so I was not worried in the least. I had the energy to do the legwork, and once I implemented my sales system, I would be off to the races.

When faced with a similar situation, always evaluate it from a distance. I knew I had to draw a distinction between strength training and cardio fitness to educate my customers on the importance of joining a health club. Lifting all day doesn't give you the health benefits of cardiovascular training, and vice versa. This distinction became an integral part of my club's sales presentation.

Furthermore, I had another unique challenge facing me: I would have to retain the loyalty of the existing members who had joined the club solely to play racquetball. When the higher-ups came in and tore out most of the courts, these people lost a place to unwind and socialize. I needed to make sure the lingering animosity was not directed at me or the new business model taking shape under their noses. I also needed this group of racquetball members on my side to help promote the new direction the club had taken. This would be my first attempt at public relations, so I did what I always do—I bought several books on the subject and started cramming.

I needed to formulate a game plan. I asked myself, what is my first step? I needed to start by surveying the club and profiling who was coming through the door and who was missing. Even though we had 12,000 square feet of newly renovated work-out floor, the majority of it was underutilized. As I said before, this company knew how to decorate a health club, and even though it was in an industrial neighborhood, it was very sellable, with a great floor plan and all of the bells and whistles: free weights, machines, aerobics, a wet area, courts, and even a small beer bar upstairs. The owners had done their job of gussying it up; now, they needed me to do my job and fill the club with members.

Back then, I had a take-no-prisoners attitude, so I put out some flyers and started interviewing for new staff immediately. The existing staff was OK, but in my mind, it was easier to train those with no experience than it was to reprogram the fixed behaviors of people who knew very little about the industry but thought they knew everything. Most of the employees had already formed alliances with each other as well as with the racquetball members, which concerned me. I didn't have time for negativity and game playing. I also thought it wouldn't hurt to bring in some new talent—in other words, pretty faces with hot, tight bodies. My hiring pattern was easy to decipher because I knew that women would attract a crowd. Here is a simple fact in life even if it isn't politically correct: get the women in the door, and the men will follow; it's just the law of nature.

Hiring pretty girls with big boobs and great butts as well as men with ripped bodies doesn't work all of the time, but when it comes to getting customers in the door fast, this strategy works most of the time. And in this case it worked extremely well because the owners could not contain their excitement when they toured the facility and saw I had not only hired fantastic brand representatives but I was also filling the club with new members much faster than projected.

I knew most of these women would not go on to become dynamite salespeople, because let's face it, it takes more than good looks to sell, but I knew with the proper training, they could get eager prospects through the door and in front of a membership contract in no time at all. For me, it was all about creating a positive emotional experience for the prospects. If the new members believed the special attention from beautiful young men and women was part of the package, they'd be ten times more likely to join and fulfill their fantasies of being healthy people surrounded by other beautiful healthy people.

Being a great manager has nothing to do with having the ability to accomplish tasks better than everyone else. Being a good or even great manager is determined by how well he or she can assemble a team of people who know how to work their strengths and are better in their fields than the manager is in that specific field. If you need a bookkeeper, find someone who loves numbers and likes to work alone; hire people who have the skill set to match the position. For example, in the club mentioned above, I needed beauty and brawn to increase traffic while I closed the sales. When you can build a team that works together seamlessly, everyone wins. Find people to fill your openings who have skills far greater than your own.

Don't be afraid to hire people who can do things better than you can. I hire salespeople for sales, trainers for training, and accountants for accounting. When I hear someone say, "I wear all of the hats," I think to myself, then you are operating in a deficit. A jack-of-all-trades is a master of none. I know there are a lot of one-man bands out there trying their best to do it all out of necessity, and I truly empathize with their situation. My tip for them is—be creative and find ways to bring professionals into their life. One way I used to get professional help when their services weren't in the budget was to barter membership(s) for the owners, employees or family members, or whatever it took to get the professional for the job. There is always a way; it is up to you to find it.

Of course, once again, it took some creative thinking to jump-start the process of growing the business. With the help of my team, I put out tons of registration boxes (a.k.a. lead boxes; I will discuss lead boxes in detail in chapter 4 and 5) and obtained a phone-and-address list of all the businesses within five miles of the club. I mailed out offers to local businesses, offering group rates for corporate memberships. I implemented an aggressive buddy-referral program to incentivize existing members to bring in their friends and relatives. I reached out to past members, who may not have known what they were missing out on, encouraging them to give us a second look and see all of the changes. I had the staff go to every business in the industrial park and give out free guest passes. We went to the local mall and gave out guest passes; we hosted a health fair, and we gave out free-tanning passes to everyone we saw. We did everything I could think of to drum up business, and it worked. We were getting a ton of daily walk-in traffic, which was unheard of for a club located in an industrial park. I even changed the club's uniform slightly to accentuate the men's muscles and the girls' curves.

Every Friday, our bar gave out a free beer to anyone who had brought a guest that week. Most men jumped on any opportunity to go upstairs to the bar because the girl tending bar was a tiny blonde with huge boobs and an even bigger smile. (As I said in chapter 1, I am not one of those guys who likes blondes with big boobs, but I didn't hire these girls for me; I hired them for the masses, and nothing sells beer like T&A.) The girls' uniforms resembled those of Hooters, except my team wore red and white, not orange and white, and wasn't near as revealing. Soon, the entire club was brimming with smiling fitness enthusiasts enjoying a rockin' club. Health clubs in the 1980s were far better than most nightclubs today because we not only had the lights and music but also swimming pools, hot tubs, exercise machines, offices, pump rooms, and massage tables, and I did my very best to use them all.

A quick funny story about this club in Kentucky: After I got the club rockin', I started enjoying my single life again. One night a couple of the members and I went out drinking and dancing. One of the girls and I decided to go back to the club for some afterhours fun. The next thing I remembered was our maintenance man saying, "Mr. Chuck, wake up! The members can see you." I looked up, and the 5:00 a.m. crowd was at the front door staring at me and my friend. The front door was glass, and the members could see straight into the aerobics room which was also all glass and unfortunately for me was where my companion and I had passed out completely naked, and were now being gawked at by a dozen early-bird members. Wow, I thought for sure I would have been canned for that stunt but yet again the owners never said a word because of the enormous success of the club. I am so glad there were no smart phones in those days.

This was the first time in my career that I thought about marketing and the necessity of advertising. Up until then, I owed my success to hitting the pavement personally and the strength of my sales system. If I could get people in the door, I could get them into a relationship with the club. Now, I was faced with the challenge of growing a business relying on corporate marketing, which, in this case, was ineffective because of the location. Corporate put a ton of marketing dollars into their flagship club, but they treated my club like an ugly stepchild. I often see this tragedy in business: an owner struggles with a club and then becomes reluctant to invest in a marketing campaign. The problem is that underperforming clubs need marketing the most. I immediately realized I was going to have to rely on my own wits, and I had a new obsession—marketing. I could no longer rely on just hard work; now, I needed to drum up leads and prospects for an entire team, not just myself. The more I thought about it, the more excited I got, and then, I had an epiphany. This was my calling in life: I would learn how to effectively market any health club in any market in the entire country. This was the answer to my question of how I would bring more value to more people. I would become the greatest marketer in the health-club industry and bring affordable health and fitness to millions while making club owners rich.

This health club was going to be my first really big success story as a guy who could take any club in any area, with limited resources, including no marketing budget, and make it a huge success. Within a few short months of moving to Kentucky to manage that club, I had quadrupled its gross income and changed the dynamics of the club forever. I eventually hired and trained a competent staff and pumped up the aerobics classes with fired-up instructors. Everyone worked as a team for the betterment of the club, and it became the place to go for fun and fitness, overcoming its less-than-ideal location. It didn't take me long to win over the old racquetball members, because I took the time to study and learn how to effectively communicate with them on their level.

This was a major turning point in my life in more ways than one, but most importantly, seeing myself succeed at assembling a great team started me on the road that brought me here, sharing my tools with you today. If it hadn't been for this early success, I may not have recognized my own need for contribution at such an early stage of my career. I needed to be a part of something bigger than myself. All the people who had helped me along the way took time out of their days to teach me everything I needed to know to get started in sales, and now, I had invaluable knowledge to share myself. I would not rest until I could harness this new knowledge and present it as a training manual for selling memberships and growing health clubs. Up until then, all of the training material was scattered; it needed to be made into a step-by-step system that could be integrated into any club's model and adapted to any salesperson's personality while still covering every scenario that might arise.

I had to learn marketing and create a marketing company that would dominate the industry, but just as I had learned the sales side of the club business, I had to learn the marketing side as well, in the real world. I needed to be in all types of scenarios, with different locations, demographics, size of clubs, budgets, business models, and price structures; my brain was going a million miles a minute. Then came the most important question we all must ask ourselves: How? How could I get hired by an owner as a club marketer when I had no idea of how to market a club or any marketing experience whatsoever? Should I go back to school and study marketing? Could I afford to go back to school? Did I want to spend three more years studying mandatory subjects when my interest was marketing and, more specifically, membership marketing? All of these questions were running through my head. I didn't have the answers yet, but I knew I would soon enough if I just kept focusing on what I wanted and not all of the challenges.

As a child, I did poorly in school because I had no interest in learning most core subjects or frame of reference as to how the subjects I was required to take would be applicable to my future. My teachers did not know how to sell students on how and why their subjects were going to be of value to us in the future. I started working at a very young age (eight years old, carrying groceries home for customers of a local store in Chicago), and ever since, I have focused on working and learning things specific to whatever job I am doing at the time. Work was far more important to me as a child because I could see the immediate return on my efforts every time I got paid.

Now, I love studying subjects like history and mathematics, as well as most subjects required by schools, but unfortunately, it took me years to learn how these subjects were applicable to my business and day-to-day life. Had I known what I know now, I might have sat up a little straighter and actually listened to a teacher from time to time, instead of using all of my energy to rebel against my formal education. I wish it would become mandatory for all teachers to take a class on selling students on their subjects. It is my opinion that students need their teachers to be evangelists of learning. If teachers could learn how to transfer their own enthusiasm about their subjects, maybe, just maybe, more students would be more engaged in their primary education.

Sales are the backbone of everything in life, from products to relationships, and people are selling every day, whether they realize it or not. You sell your kids on putting on their coats before they go outside, you sell your girlfriend on becoming your wife, you sell the plumber on fixing the sink today and not tomorrow, you sell yourself in a job interview, you sell yourself to a group of friends, and so on. We live in a world dependent on sales skills, so why not invest the time to learn how to sell effectively?

The way I saw it, marketing was just sales, but instead of selling one-on-one, a marketer sells to the masses. Then, it hit me: the way I would learn marketing (selling to the masses) was to first write a manual on the subject I knew better than any other—membership sales. This manual would then open doors to more consulting jobs, and those jobs would give me the training ground to develop my skills as a marketer. I set a goal to work with numerous health clubs throughout the United States and engineer a universal marketing campaign that could be implemented in any and every health club nationwide. It wouldn't be a cookie-cutter campaign but a universal campaign that could be tailored to the specific needs of any club yet would yield similar results in any market. I had a new purpose in life, a direction, and refueled drive, and I was ready to grab the bull by the horns.

I hated leaving the Kentucky club because I was having a blast, but it was time for me to work on my calling in life, and I needed to free up some of my time so I could write my membership-sales manual. I have always been about bringing value to the table, and it would have been unfair to the owners had I stayed on and done my job halfway while my focus was really on writing. Besides, it just isn't in me to ride the wave created by my previous success. I have to be totally committed to something, or I don't want to do it at all. The club was on its way up, and even the most inexperienced manager could go in there and maintain the growth just by showing up and letting the employees do what I had trained them to do. I needed a job where I could work minimal hours each week just to pay my bills but have no responsibilities or expectations to do anything more—and I knew the perfect club. So I moved back to my old, familiar stomping grounds and took a job as a sales counselor at the Nashville club where I started my career.

I knew there wouldn't be any questions, only open arms, and that was exactly what I needed. Besides, I was missing all my friends and my ex-girlfriend, who still worked and lived in Nashville. I had a plan and knew I could fix my working schedule to accommodate my writing schedule. No matter what, the owner, upper management, and I had maintained a great relationship. They had been good to me, and I was extremely grateful to them, and they knew it.

In the beginning, my writing took place at night and after work, because even though I was just a sales counselor, I still had a winning standard of excellence. Soon, I was down to writing every other day (on my days off). I would go to the library to work on my writing (this was before the Internet and laptops) and then later, when I got home, I would count up the few pages I had written, but it was never very many. Over the course of the first few months, I wrote only a couple of acceptable lines a day. I started to analyze all the distractions in my life to determine what was preventing me from writing at the pace I wanted. Sitting in my apartment, thinking, and knowing I had to work the next morning, I realized there were huge chunks of my day I could put to better use. Someone once told me, "If you want a new living-room set, throw out the old one. After spending a few days on the floor, you'll find a way to buy a new one." I knew it was time to get rid of the old living-room set. So once again, I resigned.

Within days of quitting my job at the club, I had a title to go along with everything I had written so far: *Job Security*. At every company meeting I had attended, at least one person inevitably complained about there being no job security in the health-club industry. I always thought to myself, if your lazy butt would learn how to sell memberships, you'd have plenty of job security. I was never a complainer, nor do I like complainers. My dad had a solution for every emotion known to man—work. If I said, "Dad, I'm bored," he'd say, "Go to work." If I said, "Dad, I'm sad," he'd say, "Go to work." My father's answer to everything was "go to work." When I was much older, I found the genius in his response. By working, you change your focus to your work and no longer feel those emotions that are holding you back because you are no longer focused on your problem. Now when I feel an uncomfortable emotion, I know exactly what to do: I go to work. Later, I used my father's wisdom and taught my employees the only path to success and job security is hard work and professional sales. I also put the words of wisdom in the most eye-catching place available—the title.

I designed a logo with a muscle head swinging a golf club, because a lot of my previous bosses preferred to be on golf courses instead of down in the trenches with their employees, selling memberships to the clubs they owned or managed. I also came up with the tagline "I drive up the gross while you drive the back nine," because I often heard my bosses say, "If I leave now, I can still get the back nine in." Including another golf reference was a way to start building up a memorable brand. In future years, I learned much more about marketing and built on the logo and tagline, as well as the golf theme, to form my marketing company, which in 1991, I named Mulligan Marketing Concepts® (or MMC® for short), which has become a trusted brand in the industry. It's the company I still manage to this day. For now, just remember to pay attention to the little things that resonate with you through your daily life, and as you accumulate these golden nuggets over time, they may become useful when it comes time for you to start your company.

Writing a health-club-sales training manual was time-consuming because I wanted to share my wealth of knowledge. By that point in my career, I had been in the health-club industry for a little more than five years. It doesn't sound like a long time, but you'd be amazed at the amount of information and education you can amass in five years if you are totally focused on a single subject, and I was. Taking chances and working with multiple clubs had served me well. I was able to test my sales systems in different scenarios and tweak them to where they could be sold as a tool with a successful track record. I continued studying everything I could get my hands on pertaining to the field of sales by reading books on topics that ranged from health and wellness to general marketing. I had so much more to say than I had originally planned, and before I knew it, I was way behind schedule.

As you can imagine, my savings ran dry, my electricity was cut, my water was turned off, and I was running out of money to buy simple necessities, like food. Shortly thereafter, the landlord put a lock on my apartment door with an eviction notice plastered there for everyone to see. This feeling was gut wrenching for me since I was raised to pay my bills and this lifestyle was in complete conflict with my values; but I knew what I was doing would change my life and the lives of millions; besides, great achievements require great sacrifices. Nothing worth having ever comes easily, and if it does, it will disappear just as easily—I guarantee it.

There are numerous perks to working in the health-club industry, and one of the biggest is being able to meet people from all walks of life. You can meet movie stars, rock stars, professional wrestlers, waitresses, and even locksmiths. So, I called up a guy I knew and told him he could have everything in the apartment except my clothes and my guitar if he could get me in. A few hours later, I moved into my new home—the back seat of my car.

Here is another piece of advice: if you are ever in a position where your next step might be sleeping in your car, try to make sure you're not doing it in the middle of the winter. But of course, only hindsight is twenty-twenty.

About a month before I got evicted from my apartment, one of my friends had come into the club where I was working and said, "Hey, Chuck, I just saw some guy drive off in your car." I ran out the door, and there was my car, going down the driveway. I asked my friend why he let the guy take my car (after all, he was a third-degree black belt and owned his own karate school), and he replied, "He had the keys; I thought you let him borrow it."

As soon as he said the guy had the keys, I knew the car had been repossessed and not stolen. I had missed a couple of payments to the guy in Kentucky whom I had bought the car from, and he had one of his friends repossess it. I wasn't angry at all; in fact, I would have done the same thing. I called him, and he confirmed my suspicion, and we worked out an arrangement for me to get the car back. I borrowed the money from my mom, and within a few days, I had my car back.

At the time, I owned a Lincoln Continental Mark V. It was a big, long white two-door coupe with dark-tinted windows and chrome spoke wheels; my friends liked to call it the Pimpmobile. For several months after being evicted from my apartment, I used the roomy interior as my new home. There was no way I was borrowing any more money for rent, because I didn't have a job, and I didn't know when I would start selling the manual. My ex-girlfriend was a champ, though, and made things bearable. She was an aerobics instructor at the club, and was still a great friend; she had even come to visit me in Kentucky when I had gotten the job there.

She was a beautiful brown-eyed brunette whose daddy was a preacher and had very little regard for me, especially after I moved into my car. Somehow, dads have a sixth sense for players like me, and they're able to sniff us out from a mile away. This girl had a rebellious streak, like many preachers' daughters (my ex-girlfriend in Knoxville was a preacher's daughter as well), and I think that's why she loved me so much. We are still friends to this day. Her parents gave her crap all the time about me, but she never let their disdain for me sway her personal opinion of me. I really did love her for that. She has a heart of gold and has been a wonderful friend over the years.

I came up with a daily routine (a system—I love systems). I went to the health club to work out and shower every morning before I started writing. As I said before, everyone knew me in the business, so I could go straight into any club around town without having to show a membership card to the club employee working the front desk. Perks—you have to love them. Then, I headed straight for the library, where I wrote until it closed. After they kicked me out of the library, I would go anywhere else I could to write until late into the evening; most of the time, I went to some fast-food joint. Later, I would find a parking lot in an apartment complex where I wouldn't be bothered by security or the police and where it was convenient for my ex-girlfriend to bring me supper from her parents' house. She stayed while I ate; then, we would make love in the back seat of the car (thank goodness for dark-tinted windows). It was funny at times how creative we had to become because I am six feet four inches tall; it was a good thing she was a contortionist. After she left, I curled up in the front seat, which was roomier, for the night. I remember some nights were so cold; it was as if I were sleeping in an icebox. Luckily, I had a big thick blanket and slept like a baby most nights. When the sun came up, my friend would be there with breakfast. I couldn't have asked for a better friend, and to this day, I value what she did for me, and I will never forget her love and kindness.

You will discover throughout this book that I am a firm believer in systems, even though I have a tendency to break rules from time to time. I have always believed in having systems to get me where I want or need to be quickly. It is necessary to break the rules once in a while, because only the rule breakers manage to separate themselves from the herd. I am a firm believer in the 80/20 rule; 80 percent of the world is either in deep debt or dead broke, so why on earth would you want to get lumped in with the majority? If you do what the 80 percent do, you'll get the same results they are getting—misery. Find your own path in life; it will be more work, but the payoff will be huge. Think outside the box, and you'll discover greatness; think inside the box, and you'll be destined to mediocrity.

For several months, this was my routine: writing, sleeping, eating, and spending time with my friend in the back seat of my car.

When I was living that life, I often wanted to just put the manual on the back burner and return to work. I knew I could get a job anywhere. Not only could I go back to work for any of the clubs I had previously worked for, but I could take over any one of the new clubs popping up on every corner. The health-club industry was exploding, and everyone wanted in on the action. Most people had absolutely no idea about the business itself, but they wanted in nonetheless. It seemed I had so many options, but I really had only one, and that was to finish the manual, stay focused on my plan, and fulfill my life's purpose. This was my destiny, and I knew it, just as I knew I was home the first time I walked into that Nashville health club; I now knew membership marketing was going to be my future.

When I finished the handwritten material (this was before laptops), I hired a lady to typeset it for me. I paid her with the little cash I had and a fake Rolex watch. While she was typesetting the manual, I took a job at a club to save up some travel money. She needed a few weeks to do her edits and typing, and then I had a couple of weeks to wait for the printing and binding of the manuals. Think about this: every time there was a minor change, I had to get in my car and drive across town to approve it. This happened several times a week throughout the process. Today, you don't even have to have printed material to start a business, write a manual, or even a book. You simply build a website and never have to leave your house. I love it!

About a month later, I had one hundred freshly printed health-club membership-sales training manuals in the trunk of my car. My goal was to travel the country, selling my manuals and learning as much about health-club marketing as humanly possible, and I would reprint manuals as needed to keep my initial costs down. But just like any good southern boy, I first had to go home and say good-bye to Mama, so I headed east down I-40 to Knoxville, Tennessee.

My mother lived in a small southern town in east Tennessee named Maryville, and as I was driving along the highway coming out of Knoxville, I noticed a big athletic club to my left. Always looking for an opportunity, I decided to stop in and practice the sales presentation I had designed to sell owners and managers on why they needed my manual and why they needed it today. I went in and asked to speak with the manager. A young guy came to the front desk and introduced himself. I spoke with him for a while and shared my enthusiasm about the health-club business and how my sales training manual had come about. He was a nice guy—not terribly knowledgeable about sales and super laid back—but a likable-enough guy. He bought a copy (the first and last copy I ever sold) on the spot; he asked me for my number, and then we shook hands and said good-bye. That evening, I received a call at my mother's house (this was also before affordable cell phones). It was the manager, and he wanted to know whether I could stop by the club the next day to meet his area director. I agreed since I was spending the night at my mother's house and would have to pass back by the club on my way out of town the following day. Besides, I was never one to pass up opportunities, and since this guy was brief over the phone, I was curious as to why they wanted to meet.

When I got back to the club the following day, the area manager was there, and we talked for a short time. I noticed the slick way he dressed and the Porsche that was undoubtedly his, parked just outside the club, almost blocking the front door. I knew immediately this was a guy who would be fun to party with because he had that mischievous look that I had seen so often from guys in the club industry. The area manager asked me whether I would mind going to their home office in west Knoxville to meet one of the owners; I agreed, and off we went. Fortunately, this was the way I was headed anyway, but at this point, I still wasn't clear as to what was on their minds.

At the office, the owner informed me he too had read the manual that morning and was hoping he could interest me in coming to work for them. He said they could offer me a good salary, a good commission structure, and a position as an assistant manager for a few months to see how things worked out, with the possibility of a general manager's position. I smiled and politely said thanks, but no thanks. I had been there and done that, but now, I was following a path to my destiny. I was nearly broke and barely had enough gas money to get me where I was going (at that point, I didn't even know where I was going—I was just hitting the road), but I still turned down the offer.

The owner and his two managers were very persistent, and I could sense they really needed my help, so finally, I said I would come on board, but only as a manager and only for the health club I had visited first (near my mother's home). I hadn't seen my mom for a while, and I thought it would be nice to spend a little more time with her before I went on the road. Plus, I knew I could rock the club in a month or two, and since the compensation package was pretty good, I would be able to save some pocket money for the road. The owner said my proposal was impossible because he would have to move or demote the present manager, which would be a radical decision since the manager had been with them for years and was the one who had brought me to the owner's attention in the first place. I thought he had a great point, and I admired his loyalty to his staff, but an assistant manager's position was not the job for me. I said it was no problem and I understood completely—thanks for the offer, but no thanks. As I was walking down the hallway to leave, the area manager came running up behind me and asked, "Please give us an hour to think of something; I am sure we can come up with something that will work for you." I agreed and told him I would get lunch and return in about an hour. I was confident that if I got the gig, I could rock the club and drastically increase membership sales within the first month, and

I could sense they knew it too because they were doing everything they could think of to keep me there. I also planned on negotiating the terms of our agreement so I would get an opportunity to review their marketing strategy and learn something from them as well.

I knew the main reason they wanted to hire me as an assistant manager was so I would be responsible for training their staff, and I was happy to do so but not as someone's assistant. I returned a short time later and they presented the idea of comanagement. They offered me a comanager's job with the same salary, commissions, bonuses, and override as the current manager.

Just in the short time I was there the day before, I knew the club was grossly underperforming, because I could see there was absolutely no fire whatsoever in the manager's personality, eyes, or heart. This club had enormous potential, so I accepted their offer, knowing full well I could add another success story to the growing list of club take-overs on my résumé.

At this time in my life, I didn't want the manager's position for the override; this time, it was to get one step closer to becoming a marketing guru. I wanted to grow the club business, and I needed to have the authority to make key decisions to implement my ideas without having to wait days or weeks for approval. I was already studying how to read people's body language, and I could read the manager very well. He was a relatively short guy and not in the best of shape; he drove a Chrysler LeBaron convertible, dressed low-end preppy, lacked confidence, was soft spoken, a little timid, and easily controlled by the area director. I knew he wouldn't get in my way, and fortunately, he was smart enough to know I was going to make him more money than he had ever dreamed of. Guys like that manager make great office workers, and owners love them because they are obedient, but they should never be put in positions to grow businesses. They lack the drive, and the worst thing you can do in business is hire the wrong people for the wrong jobs. Never try to force a square peg into a round hole.

Even though I was newly employed, I was still almost broke. I had spent all of the money I had from the previous month of work on printing and last-minute travel supplies. The club was also too far from my mother's house so I wouldn't be able to crash there; besides, I felt I was a little too old to be staying with Mama anyway. There was a roadside motel across the street from the club, which became my new home. It was dark and damp but clean and conveniently located. To move on to bigger and better things, I needed to make this club's numbers take off and take off fast; I needed to earn and earn fast. I had a few dollars but not enough to last me until the end of the month, so my brain was going full speed to think of a plan.

I went to work immediately and whipped the sales staff into shape and hired new talent, just as I had done in Kentucky. It didn't take long until we were rockin'; sales went through the roof. But as with any new adventure, there was lag time. In life, there is always a season for planting and a season for reaping. I was in the planting season at work, but my bills were in the reaping season. I had just one asset worth selling, and since I could literally walk to work, I decided to sell my car. I knew the commissions from all the membership sales would be enough to buy a reliable car on payday, but rent was due now. I was raised to always pay my bills and if possible, to pay them before they were due. This has always been one of my top priorities. Even in the toughest of times, I worked out some arrangement to pay whatever I owed. This characteristic trait has resulted in a few nights when I went to bed hungry, but at least I slept peaceful, knowing I didn't owe anyone anything. Even when I was evicted from my apartment I did everything I could to pay what I owed. I just hated to sell my car because I loved it. But as you know by now, you must be willing to make sacrifices to achieve your goals.

I ran an ad for the car in the paper and immediately started getting calls. An old guy came to my hotel and asked whether he could see the inside of the car. I kept my car spotless, and even though it was an older model, it looked better than most new Lincolns. The guy and I went for a test drive, and he loved the car. He told me he really wanted the car but was short on cash. He only had two-thirds of my asking price, but he had an old 1966 Mustang he would throw in if I would consider the deal. I said I would look at his Mustang but could not make any promises, so we drove to his house in Oakridge, Tennessee, and he showed me the car. It wasn't bad; the body was in good shape, and it ran well, but man, was it small. I wasn't a sports car kind of guy, but beggars can't be choosy, so we made the deal. I figured I could drive the car for a couple of weeks and then sell it when I got paid and add the money from the sale of the Mustang to the money from the sale of the Lincoln together to buy a newer model car. I like luxury cars, not sports cars, so I had no idea of the value of this 1966 Mustang at the time. I was just grateful that at least I had some cash in my pocket and still had a car to drive. As soon as I got back to the club, I threw a For Sale sign on the Mustang.

Not long afterward, a girl came in to ask me how much I was selling it for. I told her I really didn't know (this was pre-Google) and told her to make me an offer. She said, "I'll give you five thousand for it." I just about crapped my pants. In my mind, that Mustang was an old tiny car, and she was crazy to be paying $5,000 for a car you couldn't live in. But instead of saying what I was thinking, I said, "Show me the money!" She told me she would be back in a few days with the cash, and I said the car would be waiting, half-expecting her to come to her senses and change her mind.

Life went on, and the staff and I continued to drive up the gross in the club. Things were happening just as planned, and I was having a ball. A few days later, the girl came back with the cash and got the car. A week or so after that, it was the end of the month, which meant payday, including commissions, bonuses, and salary. I received a check for several thousand dollars to add to the five grand I got for the Mustang, plus the money I had saved from the sale of my Lincoln; so I went down to the Ford dealership and bought a sweet late-model Thunderbird. Back in those days, one of the determining factors in my car purchase was whether it was big enough for me to live in; after all, I was still going to travel the United States to learn the most effective ways of marketing a health club, which meant I had no guaranteed income or permanent residence.

At the end of the month, the club's gross sales for memberships surpassed the $200,000 mark (the majority of the revenue was on paper and would be collected over the next twelve months; it wasn't cash collected at the point of sale), and I was on cloud nine. The most that health club had ever grossed in a month was during its grand opening, and they had sold only $60,000 in new memberships. We more than tripled the sales of their very best month the first month I was there. Life was fantastic, the money was great, the women were beautiful, and I was on top of the world. Every day in that club was a party. I injected so much life into the club you could feel the energy from the highway. The members absolutely loved the experience of working out there. When guests came in, they knew they were the most important people in the world. I couldn't have been any prouder of my accomplishment. But this was never meant to be a complete chapter in my life, and just as it all fell into my lap, it was about to be just another paragraph in my past.

I heard a knock on my hotel-room door one morning. I had just woken up from a night of partying with a flight attendant who also happened to be employed by the same club as I was, which meant she technically worked for me. My comanager and the area manager were standing at the door and said the owner was at the club and would like to have a word with me. I told them I would get dressed and be over shortly. As I was closing the door, they were both breaking their necks, trying to get a peek to see who the lady sharing my bed was.

These two guys both had steady girlfriends but wanted to enjoy the perks of the business as well and envied my lifestyle. A couple of weeks before, one of the college girls who worked for us had wanted to go out with me. She was a beautiful, sexy UT student working part time, but my flight-attendant friend hated her because she was such a flirt, and she asked me not to go out with her. The flight attendant and I were never exclusive, but she was a friend, and if she disliked the girl that much, I wasn't about to hurt her feelings by following through with the date just to bang another coed, so I canceled the date. In a childish attempt to punish me, the coed slept with the comanager that night, and like a dummy, he fell in love with her immediately. I guess he had never been with a girl who was that smokin' hot before. He was so worried she was in my room that morning that he nearly broke his neck trying to see whether it was her in my bed. Had he gotten to know me, he would have known I would have never had sex with her after knowing he had hit it; friend or not, it wouldn't have been cool in my eyes.

After I got dressed, I walked over to the club and went inside. I was informed the owner, managers, and I would be meeting at the outdoor pool, where they were waiting for me. The owner started the conversation by telling me how fabulous the club was doing, and he attributed the success largely to me. At this point, I thought he was going to ask me to stay permanently and take over the area manager's job so we could grow the business company-wide, but wow, was I wrong. He continued to say the comanager setup wasn't working, and he wanted me to step down and become the assistant manager. I was flabbergasted. I admit I had a hangover, barely grasping what he was saying, but I knew this was a huge blow given what I had just done for the club. I didn't feel I deserved that, so

I told him I appreciated his position but no thanks, walked back across the street to my motel and climbed back in bed with my lady friend. Just as I was dozing off to sleep again, there was another knock on the door, with the two managers standing outside.

"Chuck, please come back. It's just a title change; your income won't be affected. Everything will be the same. Don't worry; we promise." They were saying anything and everything they could think of for me to reconsider. I don't think they ever dreamed I might resign just after making a ton of money over the past month; but they thought wrong. For me, at that point, it wasn't about the money. Had any of them studied what I taught them first about finding out what the other person wants before going into a sales presentation or negotiation, they would have known this.

I knew I brought value to a business. I knew I brought a lot to the table. I knew I was on my way to greatness. But at that time, I was completely ignorant to the importance of branding. People were still judging me for my extracurricular activities as opposed to my accomplishments. Looking back, I think I had relationships in the clubs only because I was always focused on the business; and since I was always in the clubs and recruiting new business, I was always in conversations with members; and since I focused on getting female members because I knew the males would follow, most of my conversations were with the opposite sex; and as everyone knows, opposites attract.

The clubs were filled primarily with women during the day, and I happen to love women. But never did my appetite for the opposite sex take away my focus on growing the business. In my mind, it was a win-win for me and the company. I didn't waste time on going out to dinner, lunch, nightclubs, or hotels. I enjoyed myself for a few minutes and then went straight back to growing the business-win-win, or so I thought.

The following day, when I was sober and clearheaded, I went by the corporate office to pick up my last check. The owner asked me into his office, and we had a nice funny chat about my goals but mostly about my lifestyle. I think most guys who knew me back then wished they were me but didn't have the balls for the lifestyle. He asked again whether I would reconsider. I politely told him no, that it was time for me to move on. I was never a fan of taking two steps back to gain one step forward. I was curious, though, why he made the decision to demote me after I had just rocked the club, knowing damn well the other guys would never be able to duplicate my success in a million years. He told me I was right and that he regretted his approach but not his decision. He concurred I was the best he'd ever seen at selling memberships and my sales system was far superior to anything he'd witnessed in all his years in the fitness industry, but my lifestyle was unbecoming of management. It would be easier to accept and tolerate my behavior if I were not the manager and the face of the club.

For the first time, it really sank in that no matter how great I was, people would never take me seriously if I didn't change my ways. I thanked (and admired) him for his honesty and candor. He asked me what I planned on doing, and I told him I would go out to Dallas because I read there was going to be a big health-club trade show out there in a few weeks. My plan all along was to sell copies of my manual and get some consulting jobs to work on developing some major marketing skills, and what better place to network than at a trade-show full of health-club owners? He said he had a friend who would be attending the show who had just bought into a promotional company. He said he thought I would be great at selling promotions and should give his friend a call. So I took his friend's number and thanked him for everything. After saying my good-byes to the ladies in the office I got in my T-bird, and headed west on I-40 to Dallas, Texas.

My brother lived outside of Dallas, in Mesquite, so I had a place to sleep and eat while I was out there; I was really looking forward to seeing him because we hadn't seen each other for a year or so.

I was also extremely excited about starting a new chapter of my life. I arrived about a week before the convention, so I decided to give the promoter a call and introduce myself. By this time, the Knoxville club owner had already given the promoter the low-down on me, and he was anxious to meet. We set up a meeting for the day before the show between him, his partner, and me. I knew if this was a job I wanted, I would definitely get it, and since I didn't know whether I would be moving to Detroit (where the promoter's office was) or what, I decided not to do anything until after the meeting.

I took a week off to explore Dallas with my brother, and we had a great time catching up. We went to all the sights, and it was nice not being worried about the gross sales of a club. It was the first vacation I had taken in six years and would be the last for the next twenty.

The promoter, his partner, and I met at their hotel and talked for a while. They explained their promotion to me. I had seen it run before in a health club, and knew the greatest benefit of the promotion was that it raised desperately needed cash for the owner but it had created major problems at the same time. I knew the promotion needed to be tweaked a lot to be beneficial to any health club's longevity, but the last thing I wanted to do (as a prospective employee) was to tell my future employer his program had serious flaws and needed to be fixed and I was the guy to fix it, especially in the job interview. So I listened, chimed in when appropriate, and, of course, got the job that day. There was just one hitch: they said they would call me in a week or so to finalize my move to New York (not Detroit) but only after they had closed a big deal they were in the middle of. I thought to myself, that's not a problem; I could crash at my brother's house while I waited for the call, and besides, I met a cute girl in my brother's apartment complex who I wanted to get to know better.

One week turned into two, and two weeks turned into three, until it had already been a month. I like to work, and I love to be in the middle of the action, so those weeks of waiting were torture for me. Without word from my new boss, I had to get out and find something to do. I didn't want to go to clubs to sell my manual because I didn't want to get sidetracked. After meeting with the owners of the promotion company and listening to their visions of my role in their company, I was excited about going to work for them. This opportunity fit well into my life's purpose of getting the masses interested in health and fitness via marketing. But I still loved being in health clubs and was missing the action. The twelve to sixteen-hour workdays, the highs of closing a sale, and the energy were all things I craved. So I stopped in a club from a chain I had some prior experience with and talked to the manager about some short-term employment. I was forthcoming about my situation and told him as soon as I got the call, I would have to roll. I explained I was tired of sitting on my butt all day and wanted to get back in the thick of things. He was very receptive to the idea; he was probably just excited to work with another industry guy.

He really was a health-club guy. He worked and flirted all day and then drank and snorted coke all night. Sadly, drugs were a big part of the health-club scene in the 1980s, and a lot of owners, workers, and members were indulging. Sometimes, the drugs got in the way of business and ruined people's lives and businesses, but most of the time, people were able to keep their professional lives in order. I wasn't a fan of drugs, though; my drug came in a package that was five-feet-six-inches tall or shorter, about 130 pounds or lighter, and with a great ass-piration. Other than that manager's drug and alcohol challenges, he was pretty cool. I liked him because he let me do my job and stayed out of my way. Sometimes, people forget that if they hire someone to do a job, they need to get out of the way and let him or her do it. This guy knew how to get out of the way, although I think he was just glad he could let someone else do the work for a change. His motivation didn't matter to me; I was just happy to rock!

That club in Dallas had some of the hottest female members training there. A couple of cheerleading squads from a professional sports team had memberships, and I made it a point to get to know some of them quickly. I know what you're thinking by now. You're thinking I wanted to date them, and before, you would have been absolutely correct. But after the eye-opening experience in Knoxville, I decided from that day forward I was going to keep my business life and personal life completely separate. After seeing those cheerleading squads, I thought of a great marketing idea that I just had to try out. I told the manager to ask the head office for permission to run a one-time weekend sale, allowing us to take just one dollar as a down payment on the membership (to make the contract binding) at the point of sale. The sale would run for only forty-eight hours over a weekend, and therefore, it had low to no risk. It would be the test market for a potentially enormous campaign the home office could roll out company-wide, if and when it worked. The manager thought I was nuts, but he really didn't care about much of anything anyway, so he presented it to his superiors, and the office immediately approved it.

The manager asked, "OK, now what?"

I replied, "Just sit back, and watch."

In the past, I had learned to barter for various things using health-club memberships: pizzas, clothes, hotel rooms, apartments, and so on. Here are the basics of how the barter works. You make a deal with management that you get X, and he or she gets a free health-club membership. Everyone wins because you also ask if you can put up signage and a lead box in his or her place of business (I'll discuss lead boxes in chapters 4 and 5). The club gets business from the partnering business' customers and traffic. The managers get to work out for free at the club, and they often bring in friends, who end up joining (again, the club wins), and you as the salesperson get a little perk in return. But be careful: you must preapprove all trade-outs with management first. So, I traded a dozen of these busty cheerleaders' health-club memberships in exchange for two days of casual workouts on our cardio equipment and light socializing with prospects over a two-day weekend. I put some of our cardio equipment outside in the parking lot (which happened to be on a major thoroughfare, Coit Avenue) and had these beautiful, sexy ladies demonstrate how much fun working out could be. We killed it! We sold over $100,000 gross during that weekend. To put this in perspective, Saturdays and Sundays are normally the worst days of the week for sales. These kinds of numbers had never, ever been done before in the history of the company. This was a small little gym in a strip mall. It was not at all a full-service health club. Not to mention, the club became the talk of the town—and just for the record, we signed up as many women as we did men that weekend.

A few weeks after that, my brother called me and said there was a message on his answering machine (this was pre–voice mail) saying I needed to be in New York ASAP. I called the promoter right away. He said, "We finalized the deal with three big clubs, and we need you there immediately to get the promotion set up." That was all I needed to hear. I said my good-byes to my brother, the girl I was dating, and the manager; I packed my Thunderbird and was on the road once again. I was excited about this new adventure. I was finally going to the Big Apple to take on my biggest project yet—or at least, that's what I thought.

CHAPTER 3

THE BACKBONE OF THE BUSINESS

Before I continue with the story of how I revolutionized the health-club industry, I want to give you a chapter on my sales system. Up until this point in my career, my livelihood was solely based and dependent upon this sales system, and to stay true to the chronological order of my career, I will share the system now that I used to sell thousands of memberships. Although this system was designed specifically for health-club membership sales, you can apply this system to literally any product or service. Don't get hung up on the membership label; understand with this knowledge, you can build a sales system for any product or service.

When I went to New York, my whole career changed direction. I no longer sold memberships one-on-one, but I was still in sales, which meant I kept studying the psychology, science, and data relevant to professional sales because I was now selling a much-bigger-ticket item to a more sophisticated and informed buyer. Building my sales system took thirty-five years, over a thousand books, hundreds of audio programs, countless seminars, and endless workshops, and I am still learning daily.

I am writing this book from memory, and referencing everything I've learned over the past thirty-five years would be unwieldy. Fortunately, the data (with the exception of the data needed for profiling the deconditioned market) are just a few key strokes away. I am not claiming I discovered all of this information. Quite the contrary—eighty percent of the things in this book have been said a thousand times before in a thousand different formats and in a thousand different ways from a thousand different authors. I did the research and then painstakingly molded it piece by piece into this system that is tailored specifically, for health-club membership sales.

Please do not skip this chapter, because whether you are in sales as a profession or not, you are still selling something in life every day, and what's even cooler than learning how to sell is knowing how and when someone is selling you so you can always come out on top.

I was hesitant to put this chapter in the book because over the years, I have seen many articles and books authored by people using bits and pieces of my sales system, claiming it as their own. I say this only because I don't want to confuse you, the reader, as to who is the true architect of this sales system. But the more I thought about it, the more I realized this is an educational book, and I want to share everything with you, especially if it can change your life, and learning to sell effectively will definitely change your life. This chapter will give you the tools to sell any health-and-fitness product, including health-club memberships. Most of the material you'll read or learn from other companies is only the basics that I have either published or put on MMC®'s website, in videos, blogs, vlogs, text content, and so on. These companies that "borrow" my information normally stick to the talking points and rarely go into any depth since the information hasn't been available to them until now. But now, I am going to take you deeper than ever before so you'll know far more than the "experts."

Earlier, I told you when I was in Nashville around 1985, I was interviewed by a local newspaper about the health-club industry. I shared the basics of this system with them for the article; later, in May 1999, I wrote an article for *CBI* (*Club Business International*) magazine titled "Sales Specifics," where I shared even more of my sales system. I was asked to speak on the same subject matter at the following IHRSA (International Health, Racquet, and Sportsclub Association) convention later that year in Orlando, Florida, where again I spoke on this subject matter. I have taught the basics of my sales system to over a thousand health-club owners and thousands upon thousands of health-club employees. I have had the basic portion of this sales system on MMC®'s website since December 12, 1999. I started giving a condensed version of this sales system free as a download and continue to give it today as a free download on our new and improved website, healthclubmarketingmmc.com, along with tons of free marketing tips, blog posts, vlogs and videos, in an attempt to teach people how to grow their health-and-fitness businesses. In short, I have been sharing the online portion of my system with thousands and thousands of people since its conception in 1985. However, today, you will learn the never-before-released portion of this system in this book, so be prepared to earn your PhD in professional sales.

I was extremely fortunate because I learned my profession in the natural order it should be learned: sales and then marketing. You must first be well versed and have a proven track record of success in one-to-one sales, or it is highly unlikely you will be able to effectively market a club or handle the responsibility of growing a business. If your closing percentage is not at least 80 percent, focus 100 percent of your time on this chapter, in which I will teach you a professional sales system that you can apply to any business, product, service, or industry. I spent five years in the trenches with 100 percent of my time devoted to honing my craft before I even considered going to the next phase of learning—marketing. Then, I spent the next five years honing effective marketing skills, bringing behind the other five years, before I ever felt confident I knew what I was doing. There are no shortcuts, but there are accelerated learning tools, and in this chapter, I eliminate the BS and teach you exactly what you need to know to sell health products and health-club services. I have done the research for you, I have done the travel, I have invested the money, and I have been the one to put everything on the line, and now, I have put it all into this book for your consumption—Bon appétit.

I am a firm believer in giving value, and since you parted with your hard-earned capital to buy this book, I want to ensure you receive enormous value. So, I am going to give you the details of this professional sales system, and then you can go to our website, healthclubmarketingmmc.com, and get the free download; now, you will have my entire system, which I have been updating every year since the early 1980s. Throughout this chapter, I will reference some of the forms pertinent to this system, but since you can get them off our site, print ready, I don't want to take up valuable space in this book. I prefer to fill it with more detailed information to teach you the psychology, social sciences, and data that are the behind-the-scenes tools used to create this system, so you too can custom-design a sales system for any health-and-fitness product or service (or any product or service you choose).

The three S rule—sales, service, and sanitation (previously mentioned in chapter 2) is a highly debated subject as to which comes first (because they are equally important) with fitness fanatics (similar to the chicken or the egg). Some fitness fanatics are delusional about business and still believe in the *Field of Dreams*: if you build it, they will come and they will automatically buy. Well, part of that delusion is correct; if you build a beautiful new facility, with all the bells and whistles, and have the latest equipment, people will come and check you out. Most people are curious by nature and love to see new shiny things. But that's where the fantasy falls apart, along with most new owners' dreams. Consumers have more options today than ever before, and what's more, they have access to them on their gadgets. Most prospects don't even have to walk in your club to check you out. They simply go online and see everything you have to offer from the comfort of their homes. Owning a brick-and-mortar business today is tough. We need prospects to come in the door so their senses can be engaged with the product.

Sales and salespeople have gotten a bad reputation over the years because of a few bad apples, but I guarantee you this country, your state, your business, your home, and your lifestyle all have a salesperson who made it happen. Everything you love has a sale behind it. I am married now, with four kids ages nine through thirteen, and every day, I am faced with some of the best salesmanship I've ever seen. When my kids (especially my third son, Coley) want to go somewhere or do something, they turn on the sales charm; when my wife wants something, she knows how to get me to say yes. All people are selling themselves daily, to their spouses, parents, coworkers, friends, relatives, bosses, kids, and so on. Anytime you want something or want to get your way, you are in a sales presentation.

Think about it: there are a ton of great products sitting in warehouses that have never made it to consumers because no one effectively sold those products to the public. How many great musicians, writers, actors, inventors, and so on do you know who never made it because they didn't try (or know how) to sell themselves? On the other hand, look at the most successful people in the world, and I guarantee they are salespeople. Steve Jobs and Bill Gates are thought of as tech guys, but these billionaires are greater salesmen by far. Bill sold his software to IBM, and Steve sold Apple to the world. A sale takes place when one person transfers to another his or her enthusiasm about a product, a service, an idea, a dream, a marriage proposal, or a night at a friend's house—literally anything and everything you can think of.

So, if you know salespeople shape the world, and you want to shape the world, why not become the best damn salesperson ever? If you have the heart, I guarantee that you will obtain the tools in this chapter. I cannot stress how important it is for you to learn how to sell yourself, your club, your products, and your services, if you want to have any success whatsoever. So, whether you are selling training equipment, tanning beds, supplements, boxing equipment, food and beverages, massages, personal-training sessions, classes, and so on, you will be able to use this system. Also, if you are just a health-and-fitness enthusiast, you will learn all the techniques salespeople are using when you buy a product or service, including a health-club membership, which will give you the upper hand and save you thousands of dollars in membership fees. So, let's get started.

"The person with the most information and knows how to use that information wins the negotiation." (Chuck Thompson).

The first thing you need to do is get in the right state of mind before going to work and definitely before going into a sales presentation. Just as athletes warm up before practice or a game, you need to warm up before taking calls or presenting guests. Shit happens, and we all know that, so let's be prepared. There are going to be days when everything seems to be going wrong, and the last thing you want to do is go into a presentation or speak on the phone when you are not in the zone.

Avoid the three *H*'s: hot, hungry, or horny. People get aggravated, irritated, and impatient when they are hot or hungry, and people lose focus when they are horny (or maybe that's just me— whoops, TMI). So, make sure you eat a good healthy breakfast before work, dress comfortably but appropriately, and the third *H*, well, that is in your hands—no pun intended.

Here are ten exercises and things you can do to prepare yourself for the day and for your presentations:

1. Questions: Every morning, I ask myself a series of questions to get focused on the things that are really important to me so I have a clear direction for the day. You may not be conscious of it, but you ask yourself hundreds of questions daily, both good and bad. It is up to you to design questions that will serve you and not hurt you.

For example, ask yourself, who am I going to help today? Whose life will I change today? How can I make this the best day ever?

Don't ask questions like, why do I have to work today? When am I going to get what I want in life? Why is my neighbor more successful than I am?

Your brain can only answer the questions you ask it, so choose your questions wisely and design your questions so you'll get the answers that will empower you and not depress you—you're the programmer.

Ask yourself questions like these before you go into a presentation: If I don't do my very best for this prospect, how much will it cost me and him or her? How can I make this prospect realize that this is the club where he or she will get the best results? If I half-ass this presentation and skip steps, will I regret it later? If this prospect leaves this club today without making a commitment, will he or she join my competitor just because I was too lazy to give my very best?

The reason you want to ask yourself great questions is because your brain (which is the most powerful computer in the world) will search for (or directs its focus toward) an answer for the empowering questions. When you are faced with a challenge, you should always ask yourself what is great about this, how you can turn it around to be a valuable tool, and so on. You have the most advanced computer resting on your shoulders with the fastest search engine known to mankind. Start using your computer more effectively by asking yourself empowering questions and focus on what you really want.

2. Posture: The way you carry yourself will affect your attitude. Make sure you stand tall, with your shoulders back and your head straight; you are a winner, and winners walk, talk, and carry themselves like winners. Strike the victory pose: put your arms above your head as if you just won the gold, and hold it for sixty seconds. Studies on this pose suggest it really does boost your confidence.

3. Visualization: Imagine going through the day, and everyone is smiling and laughing, and you're in control. You are closing every sale, everyone is patting you on the back, you are the envy of everyone, and every new member is leaving your office knowing they had just made the best decision of their life. Create this image in your mind, because your brain doesn't know the difference between what has actually happened and what you are just imagining. Top athletes are known to use this visualization technique in preparation for competition; if Olympians use this technique, you should too.

4. Affirmations: Affirmations are words that you chant over and over to yourself and are said with positivity, intensity, and varying tonality. For example, you can say, "I am the greatest salesman in the world," "I am a winner," "I always win," or something like, "I am a lean, mean, fighting machine" (from an old Bill Murray film). The idea is to come up with your own affirmations from your heart that motivate you, and say them throughout the day with intensity and conviction.

5. Breathing: Everyone living is breathing, but not everyone knows how to breathe properly. There are a couple of breathing exercises you should be aware of. I learned them in martial arts, and they have a calming effect. First, I take deep breaths as I limber up my body in a tai chi sort of way: I take a deep breath in, hold the breath, and then exhaling as I change my stance, either pushing out, up, or down with my hands. The other is to take in four short, fast breaths and exhale four short, fast breaths.

6. Focus: I get perturbed when I hear the label "genius" thrown around. We can all be geniuses if we just have unwavering focus on any given subject, task, field, endeavor, and so on. People say Michael Jackson was a musical genius; I disagree. I believe people like Michael Jackson, Michael Jordan, and Stevie Ray Vaughan are totally focused on their goals and put every ounce of their energy and minute of their days into perfecting their love for music,

sports, arts, business, sales, marketing, and so on. Focus on your goals, and you can become a genius too.

7. Smile and laugh often: Laughing puts you in a good mood. It is impossible to be sad or angry when you are laughing or smiling. People tend to mirror others, and when you smile, most people will smile back. A simple smile can change your future as well as the quality of your life.

8. Humming: Hum a familiar tune to eliminate fear. Humming distracts the analytical part of your brain, which helps you stop thinking for a minute to clear your head. Also, if you feel nervous, remember to hum for sixty seconds before your presentations; you'll forget you are nervous.

9. Calming yourself: A sale is a performance, and the last thing anyone wants to witness is a performer with performance anxiety. You must be in control and confident at all times. One way to calm your nerves is to carry something in your pocket or in your hand that is familiar and comforting. It will calm you and soothe your nerves. It's just like a child with a security blanket.

10. Attire: Always dress for success, which translates into always dress for your prospects. People like people who look (or dress) like they do. This was very hard for me early in my career when I started consulting because I dressed super smooth. *Miami Vice* was a show in the early 1980s, where they dressed really sharp, and I absolutely loved the look and wore it well; then in the late 1980s Nike came out with a line of Michael Jordan warm-up suits which were super cool too and I wore Jordan head to toe, but club owners were more conservative dressers, which meant that later in my career, I came to love khakis, button-downs, golf shirts, and blue blazers. So before you leave the house, think of your customers, and dress for them, not for yourself. Again, learning the balance is the key to dress to impress. Never overdress or underdress. Do your best to mirror your prospects or at least your industry.

Once you get to the club, prepare your office for success. Turn your computer on, and clean your desk of clutter. Have the files that are relevant to the day's tasks and appointments on your desktop and nothing else. Make sure your office is clean and neat. Cleanliness is extremely important, and that goes for your body, breath, clothes, and office. People who present themselves sloppily will convey that message to their prospects.

Put a couple of pictures on the wall that are relevant to your goals—health-and-fitness models or inspirational messages. But only have a couple; make sure they are not too busy, and keep them on the wall behind you, so the attention of your guest will always be forward.

Colors matter; they trigger different thoughts, feelings, and emotions, so learn how to use them to your advantage. The color green is comforting and relaxing. Green signifies that food and water are readily available and relaxes us. I am not a fan of the color green, but I'll use any tool available to me to close a sale. The color of success is red. Red is a powerful color and draws people to you. Red makes you stop and pay attention. Ladies, if you want more attention from men, wear red. They will definitely stop and take notice. The color blue is thought to enhance our creativity and is linked to hygiene, water, and purity. Yellow is believed to trigger hunger. This is why most fast-food restaurants have yellow in their logos.

Always offer the prospect something warm, like hot tea or coffee; if the prospect is holding something warm, it will help him or her warm up to you. Getting your prospect to feel positive sensations in your presence is paramount to your success. The three most powerful sensations are warmth, softness, and weight:

- Warmth links our brains to security; yes, a simple cup of coffee or a hot cup of tea can send this sensation to the brain. Now the prospect will begin to let his or her guard down and trust you more.

- Softness is a great way to soften your prospects up to be influenced. Get two soft chairs for your office for prospects to sit in, and make sure your chair is hard. People who sit in a hard chair are much tougher negotiators, and since you want to be in charge, don't let yourself get too comfortable.
- Weight is associated with the feeling of quality. Later when you take the prospect on a tour of the club, you'll get the prospect on the equipment so he or she will experience this sensation as well.

Now that your office is set up properly for conducting business, start calling to confirm your appointments for the day. The calls should be short and sweet. If the prospect doesn't answer the phone, it is OK to leave a voice mail or send a text message. The call should go something like this: "Hey, Chuck, this is Bob from ABC Athletic Club. I just wanted to call and let you know that if you want to bring someone with you for your workout (or to visit our club), you are more than welcome to. I look forward to seeing you at four p.m. today. Thanks, and have a great day." Say nothing negative; your words should all be positive. You also could say, "I just wanted to remind you to bring your towel," or anything else, just to get him or her committed to the appointment.

Today's membership directors have it much easier with e-mails and text messages, because if you can get the prospect to agree to an appointment in writing, he or she is far more likely to show up for the appointment than if the confirmation was verbal. So, use these tools when possible, and have your prospects confirm by e-mail or text message so they are more committed to the appointment.

You must know how to answer the phone properly, handle an information call, and do a proper handoff—turn the guest over to the membership director (a.k.a. sales counselor or a salesperson).

These three steps are covered in the free download on my website; so make sure you go to healthclubmarketingmmc.com.

I have divided my sales system into three key parts: interview, tour, and close. I believe most presentations last about an hour, so I want you to think of each section as a twenty-minute session. They say people's minds start to wander after twenty minutes of doing the same task, and since the goal is to keep our prospects engaged, try to keep each portion to no more than twenty minutes. Of course, there are always exceptions to any rule, and if your prospect is fully engaged, don't worry about the time.

In the interview, you want to probe and ask questions. The more questions you ask, the more information you will have, and as you now know, the person with the most information (and knows how to use that information) always wins. This holds true in just about everything in life but especially in sales. The questionnaire flow is paramount, so do your best to keep the prospect in one mind-set at a time. If at all possible, complete all of your questions about a specific topic before moving on. Ask the easy questions first. Save sensitive questions for the end when you have already built a rapport with the guest. Try to set up your questions so they flow from one to the next seamlessly. Probe for problems, and magnify the pain that has been caused by being overweight or out of shape, such as health issues and stamina.

Start looking for signs of the prospect's preferred communication. Is it visual or auditory? Prospects who are visual communicators use their hands a lot. Prospects who are auditory communicators speak loudly, quickly, and with inflections. Learn to speak at the proper pace when presenting, especially when presenting to an auditory communicator. It is said that you should speak at a pace of about three-and-a-half words per second to get the best results. If you speak too slowly, you'll sound condescending or slow minded, and if you speak too fast, you risk coming across as untrustworthy. You will see their preferences as you dig deeper into their feelings and emotions during the interview. Once you nail down their preferred way of communicating, start to align with your prospects by using their preferred way of communicating. People like people who are like them. Care enough to enter into their world.

You also want to determine which social style your prospect has. Is he or she a director, a relator, an analytic, or a socialist? The reason why these are so important to understand is because everyone falls primarily into one of these categories, but people do not follow any specific social style 100 percent. For example, your core social style may be a director, but as a director, you still have some of the traits of a socialist, a relator, and an analytical.

It's important to understand these four social styles because each prospective member you engage in a sales presentation is going to fall into one of them. The more you know about each social style, the better equipped and prepared you will be to accommodate that prospect. One of the first things we learn as children is the Golden Rule: "Treat others the way you want to be treated." I have changed this because I believe you should treat others the way *they* want to be treated.

What I mean by this is if you are speaking with a prospect whose core social style is a director, and you approach him or her with a socialist social style, the prospect is going to be annoyed because he or she wants you to get straight to the point and not socialize. The same goes if you are trying to lock up a relationship with a socialist; if you approach him or her as a director—straight to the point—the prospect is going to perceive you as being rude and unfriendly and therefore will be annoyed by your approach, making it less likely he or she will want to enter into a relationship with you and your health club. When you adjust your personality to theirs, you are not being a phony; you are paying the prospect the highest compliment possible by demonstrating you care enough to enter into their world.

Throughout the years of studying the psychology of sales and marketing, I have heard several different variations of this concept of four social styles, and there are numerous labels for each style, depending on the psychologists you are listening to or the book you are reading. I, however, prefer to look at them as the four basic personality types. Again, forget the label because all that matters is you are familiar with them as well as their strengths and weaknesses. Below are brief descriptions of the four types.

A director is straight to the point, wants the bottom line, does not waste his or her time, is very impatient, and may come across as arrogant and self-centered.

The analytical wants the numbers, the details, as well as anything and everything to review; analytical people are normally middle of the road, with few highs or lows.

A socialist loves to socialize. Relationships are extremely important. He or she is a flashy dresser, loves bright colors, has pictures everywhere, and is typically not very organized.

A relator needs to relate to others. He or she considers what everyone else thinks, never wanting to upset the norm, and finds it difficult to make decisions on their own.

Another great marketing tool is to use the prospect's name as much as possible because we associate positive feelings with our names, and our brains light up when hearing our names.

The power of eye contact is important as well. Direct eye contact is a tactic for dominance and commands authority. Staring, on the other hand, scares people and makes them uncomfortable, which goes back to the predatory fears of our past. If you are uncomfortable with eye contact, look just above the center of the other person's eyes. It looks as if you are looking straight into a person's eyes, but you're not, which will be comforting to you.

Interview

The interview is your time to listen and ask your prospect questions. This is not a time for you to make suggestions, tell your story, give advice, or have any other dialogue. Let the guest talk. Remember, people's favorite subjects are about themselves, their families, their pet projects, and so on. Use this time to get as much information as possible. Your ability to conduct a proper interview will be the key to your success not only in this area of your business but in all aspects of your life. We were born with two ears and only one mouth; our creator was trying to tell us something. As in most things, the foundation must be strong enough to build upon. The interview is the foundation of the membership sale and it must be strong enough to support you through each additional phase, all the way to the end of your presentation.

It is imperative you interview guests before you tour them around the club. How else will you know exactly what their interests are? And equally important, how will you know where to start and end your tour? Most novices start the presentation with the tour, which is ignorant because the tour needs to be designed around the prospect's wants and needs. Another huge mistake is to have a canned tour. Every tour must be tailored to the prospect's emotions, wants, needs, and social style. Never tour anyone without first sitting down somewhere quiet and conducting a proper interview.

Before you even start an interview with a prospect, you have to remember certain things: The interview portion is about asking prospects how they feel about health-and-fitness, your health club and its products and services. Understanding the role psychographics play in the decision-making process and therefore uncovering important attitudes, perceptions, beliefs, and behaviors are extremely important to be more effective in locking up the relationship. You want to gather as much information about the prospect sitting in front of you as possible and know exactly what it is that triggered him or her to come into your health club today. What emotions are driving the prospect to the club? Everything you want to know about a prospect can be discovered in the interview. If you uncover the pertinent information that is necessary, you will lock up the relationship and have a new member.

Your primary goal is to get the prospect to associate as much pleasure as possible with being a member of your club and associate even more pain with not making the commitment today. But first, you must unearth the prospect's goals, needs, and wants. Show the prospect you truly care, and emphasize your concern for the prospect's goals. You should show all prospects that you are committed to helping them achieve their goals, and all this can be accomplished through a properly executed presentation starting with an interview.

I have designed an interview questionnaire called the "Tour Sheet" to discover guests' goals, wants, likes, and dislikes so you can show them how your club, product, or service can fulfill their needs and wants. I call the interview questionnaire a tour sheet to remind the sales representative to ask the questions first before taking the guest on the tour of the property. This way the professional salesperson can use the answers as a guide as well as a reminder of the guest's interests throughout the tour. If you haven't downloaded the tour sheet yet, do it now at healthclubmarketingmmc.com. In the download, I cover the tour sheet in detail, so I'll just hit the highlights in this book to save room for information that isn't covered in the download.

The tour sheet (questionnaire) serves three purposes:

1. Learn enough about guest to guide him or her on the correct path to achieve their goals.
2. Uncover and be prepared for their probable objections.
3. Gather the right information to help guests make an emotional buying decision today.

Here are the four core objections you'll hear when trying to lock up a relationship with a prospective member:

1. *Time*—I don't know whether I have the time.
2. *Money*—I don't know whether I can afford it.
3. *Spouse*—I need to speak with my spouse before making a decision.
4. *Think about it*—I need more information.

Since you are now well aware of the core objections before they even arise, it is up to you to prepare in advance for them. All four of these objections can easily be overcome with logical and emotional reasoning. To overcome these objections, you simply have to ask the right questions and secure the appropriate answers before the objections are even verbalized. There are unlimited objections, but these four are the core objections. I have seen people try to replace one or two of these to pass my system off as their own, replacing them with things like weather or location. Location is an objection that may come up once every one hundred times because most prospects who visit your club, or whom you are targeting with your marketing, either live or work in the area. Weather, on the other hand, is absurd. The busiest month of the year for health clubs in the United States is January. It is poor weather that drives most fitness enthusiasts inside for their exercise. Maybe in other countries, weather is a core objection but in the United States it is rarely an issue. By the end of this chapter, you will be prepared for any objection in any country and have the tools to overcome them all.

Build rapport with your prospects because people buy products they associate the most pleasure to as well as the person they feel the most connected with. The same principle applies to pain; people do not buy products they associate with pain (dislike) or from a person they associate with pain or are even just uncomfortable with.

Start building a rapport with the prospect first before you explode with enthusiasm; later, you will know how to express your enthusiasm once you determine the type of prospect you have in front of you and have gauged their level of enthusiasm. You can't start at level ten if your client is at level one; you'll blow him or her out of the water. The same is true if he or she is at level ten, and you're at level one; you'll bore the prospect to death. Find common denominators, and align with the prospect. People like people who are like them or are how they want to be. When people are not similar to each other, they tend not to like each other. If you find yourself in a situation where you don't immediately like a prospect, ask yourself what you could like about him or her. Align first with the prospect; then, lead the prospect.

You must know your product well and be enthusiastic about it and its possibilities, but pace yourself to first gauge your prospect. Building rapport is the easiest part of the presentation; the best way to build rapport is to find a common denominator between you and the prospect. Health and fitness are obviously two common denominators, but they are just the beginning. Don't stop there; find more common denominators to make a tighter connection. Other ways of building rapport are to give a sincere compliment, find a common interest, tell a relevant story, and so on. Connect and become his or her best friend. The prospect wants to know whose interests you are really paying attention to: his or her interests or your commission. Remember, the Golden Rule is wrong. You should do unto others as *they* would have you do unto them. Building rapport is about the other person, and in sales, your feelings don't matter; the prospect's feelings are all that matters.

Learn the art of mirroring. Mirroring builds rapport by getting two people to feel the same emotions. Neurons light up in your brain when you mirror someone or he or she mirrors you, which means we feel what we see—a connection. Engage prospects on their level; use their vocabulary, body language, preferences of communication, and social style. Mirroring communicates that you are on the same page, from the same tribe. This goes back millions of years. If someone was different, the members of the tribe were afraid he or she would compete for their resources, but when he or she was the same as other members of the tribe, everyone tended to relax and get comfortable.

Try using some of these questions to start building rapport:

1. How is your health right now?
2. How does current health compare to last year?
3. What are your goals for this year?
4. Are you on track to meet your goals?
5. How do you feel right now about your fitness level?
6. At what age did you feel the most fit in your life?

Questions are the greatest friends of a salesperson. By far one of the most important skills that separate professional salespeople from novices is knowing when and how to ask questions. Questions help get to the deeper levels of attitudes and feelings, they also can bring thoughts and ideas to the surface that aren't easily or quickly expressed. A professional salesperson can probe deeper into every answer the prospect gives by turning it into another question. Probing is learned through trial and error and is best done by feel. When you ask some very simple questions, you will uncover unmet needs, wants, wishes, desires, and then you can present a way for the prospect to meet them and take the presentation to the next level.

It is important you completely understand the principles of pain and pleasure as they relate to people's choices. Everything we do in life boils down to two driving forces: the desire to avoid pain and the desire to gain pleasure. Whether subconsciously or consciously, you are either moving toward pleasure or away from pain. The clothes you wear, the car you drive, the clubs you join, the friends you have, and even things as small as the way you comb your hair are all guided by your association with the pain or pleasure it will bring you.

Unfortunately, people will do far more to avoid pain than they will to gain pleasure. But it is imperative you learn ways to motivate your prospects by using either force. Ask yourself this: Do you tend to do things because it's crunch time (your butt is on the line), or do you tend to jump right in and get things done based on the possibilities (goals and sense of achievement)? If someone tends to wait to the last minute, he or she is likely pain-motivated; and if the person tends to jump right in and get things done immediately, he or she is likely pleasure-motivated. Your goal is to stimulate the prospect's wants, wishes, goals, and desires and to stir up the prospect's pain of not making a change today, while linking enormous pleasure to making a decision today. This is known as the carrot-and-stick method of motivation. Ask the right questions, and you'll easily determine which method of motivation your prospect responds to more favorably and be able to shape your presentation around that method.

You should have two types of questions prepared—one set to stir up pain and another set to stimulate pleasure, evoking positive emotions toward your product and services.

Here are some examples:

- Pain: Are you currently in the best shape of your life?
- Pleasure: When were you the happiest with your fitness level, health, and appearance?

I assure you there was a time when the prospect felt awesome, sexy, and full of energy; you just need to discover when and bring it to the surface so he or she can relive the time and experience those feelings now. Think of it this way; isn't there certain songs that take you back to a certain time, place and memory in life that evoke certain emotions and feelings? It's a rhetorical question, of course there are. It is your job to take the member back in time whether it was yesterday or twenty years ago and get them to feel those same feelings and emotions right now and link those positive feelings and emotions to your product. The beautiful thing with this technique is that you are the conductor and can chose which feelings and emotions to evoke by the questions you ask.

An undisturbed prospect will not buy your products or services today. Unearth desires that are not being met and pleasures that have been suppressed. Paint a mental picture of exactly what he or she wants, and show him or her the possibilities. Get the prospect to focus on the positive and make it real. Ask more questions, such as, "If you did achieve your goals in less than three months, would you be happy again the way you were back then? How would that make you feel?" Get his or her imagination to start seeing the mental picture (make it real). Then, go back to that throughout the presentation—for example, say something like, "Just picture your perfect body." Whatever someone is thinking about, he or she will feel the emotion associated with that experience. For example, "Tell me about the time when you felt the happiest in life. How did it feel? What were you doing?" Now, he or she will start to feel those same feelings. The same principle applies to sadness. Whatever we focus on, that's what we will feel.

Here are a few more sample questions to stimulate pleasure and stir up pain. These questions evoke pleasure:

1. What is it exactly that you would like to accomplish in the next thirty days?
2. What part of your life would you change if you could?
3. What would it take for you to love training?
4. What do you want to get out of being a member of our health club?

5. If money were not an issue, what would you want out of life?
6. Where do you want your health to be five years from now?

And these questions bring up pain:

1. What will happen if you don't join today?
2. How will you feel if you miss out on this opportunity?
3. Have you failed yourself in the past?

Now that you have started to stir up the prospects' pain, it is time to relieve them of their pain by demonstrating how your club, product, or service will eliminate all of their pain and frustration and have them enjoying their lives, full of energy and feeling all of their past pleasures once again, in just a few short months.

The interview should take about twenty minutes as I said in the beginning, but do not proceed to the tour until you have the prospect emotionally engaged. If you need more time, take it because this is where you need to have the prospect selling themselves on why they must join today. It is very important to reiterate that prospects buy for emotional reasons and justify their purchases with logical reasons, so make absolutely sure you have enough emotional reasons to justify the prospect joining today before going to the next phase.

Tour

The tour is the time to demonstrate how your club has everything needed to achieve the prospect's goals and transfer your enthusiasm to your prospect. Demonstrations always grab people's attention and create interest. Always carry a pen and paper or a tablet (refrain from using your mobile to avoid looking unengaged) with you so you can take notes of your prospect's answers and responses, as well as your observations. You only retain 20 percent of the information you hear and 40 percent of the information you hear and see, but if you hear, see, and write down the information, your retention goes up to 80 percent.

Always start the tour with the prospect's area of least interest and end in the area of his or her greatest interest—build up to the climax. Remember after the tour is done, it's time to do the paperwork (close the sale), and you want the prospect enthusiastic when you start to fill out the paperwork. Always end on a positive note, because the prospect will remember the last part of the tour and conversation more than the beginning or middle; this phenomenon is called the recency effect.

Whatever you do, make sure your statements and facts are consistent throughout your presentation as well as consistent with those of your coworkers. It's called the consistency principle. When a person hears things that are consistent, his or her brain releases dopamine (the pleasure chemical), making the person feel happy. However, inconsistency suppresses dopamine, which produces negative feelings. Inconsistency makes us very uncomfortable. In our evolutionary past, inconsistency was very bad, and people who were inconsistent were deemed untrustworthy and therefore shunned by the tribe. Our brains developed a way to punish us for being inconsistent. That is why you must always be consistent with your message. It is so deeply rooted in our brains that it will always be a game changer.

The same goes for repetition. People believe a familiar statement after they have heard it at least three times. But don't say it exactly the same way each time; convey the point in three different ways while still saying the same thing. We need consistency in our lives. So, design some great statements about your club, and say them consistently throughout the tour.

It is extremely important to involve the prospect's five senses (sight, hearing, touch, smell, and taste) during the tour. This will get him or her more connected with the club and therefore more excited about becoming a member, which will make your job far easier. The sale is made during the interview and on the tour, if you learn how to profile your prospect, for example, communication preference, social style; ask all the right questions to stimulate pleasure, stir up pain, and get the prospect's senses involved throughout the tour; the closing of the sale will be just a formality of doing the paperwork.

You must get prospects on the equipment; take them into a group class, whether it's a spinning class, aerobics class, or any other class. It doesn't matter as long as it's high energy and members are having fun. Get prospects to step in the sauna or steam room, feel the temperature of the pool, smell the fat-free muffins in the juice bar, meet the trainers, meet some members, hold racquets in their hands, hit tennis balls, anything and everything that gets their senses engaged—no excuses, just do it. The retail industry spends millions of dollars to learn consumers' buying patterns, and they know better than anyone that if they can get you to touch a product, you'll probably buy it.

Here is an important note about smell: When a salesperson tries to sell you something and has bad breath, or is wearing an obnoxious amount of cologne or perfume, do you buy from him or her? Smell is one of the fastest things that can change a state of mind, for example, take you from being interested to being disgusted. When you are an infant, your sense of smell develops before most of your brain develops. Some smells trigger the emotion of disgust (one of the most powerful emotions), and when a prospect is disgusted, game over.

In many instances people buy based on the emotions and feelings the product will give them, not because of the product itself. If you are excited about a product and convey (transfer) that excitement, the prospect will want those feelings of excitement as well. People will buy whatever the product or service is, provided the product or service can produce the same feelings or emotions.

When we feel pleasure, we want to experience it often. The feeling of familiarity takes over and makes us feel good. You must be able to transfer your enthusiasm about health and fitness as well as your club to your clients.

Be very careful if you have any unresolved concerns or doubts about your product or any aspects of your product, because you are certain to unconsciously convey them to the prospect. You better resolve these issues before meeting with any potential members. I once read if you are mad, worried, confused, or in any other negative state of mind or feeling any negative emotions when thinking about your product or service, you will associate those same feelings with that product or service. The opposite is also true; if you are happy, excited, enthusiastic, and so on, you will associate positive feelings with your product or service. When you talk about your product negatively to your spouse or coworkers, you'll link negative thoughts to your product. In some cases, people do this so often they can never sell the product again.

When a prospect starts to focus on negatives or untruths, carefully align with the prospect ("I understand your concerns") and then redirect them to the positives ("let me show you what we have found"). Make absolutely sure before you go on a tour you are fully prepared to project the exact feelings you must convey to get the desired results. Get your mind focused on the good things in your life, about your products and services, and the club. It is imperative you are 100 percent confident and enthusiastic when it comes to your product and services.

As you are touring the club, ask a series of questions, but be sure to allow the prospect time to expound on his or her answers. When you are asking questions, learn to pace the questions so they don't turn the tour into an interrogation. Below are lists of questions to stir up positive and negative emotions during the tour. I am just giving you a few examples; feel free to rewrite them using your own words, context, and delivery. You should subtly ask your questions throughout the tour; be patient and make sure you come across as truly interested, and don't let the questions seem intrusive.

Put together some yes questions (questions you know will be answered with a yes) to get some smaller yeses to build up to the big yes later in the closing; this is called the foot-in-the-door (FITD) technique. Ask easy yes questions first, like "Isn't it a beautiful day?" And start working your way up to the big yes, which will be "Yes, I want the membership to start today."

Below are some of the core emotions that will always play a role in your sales presentations, so learn how to use them to your advantage. Design as many questions as you can think of to evoke these emotions.

The following list are some negative emotions we all feel from time to time which can be used to motivate prospects to make a buying decision today:

- Fear: People are naturally afraid of being left out. Capitalize on this fear, and show prospects that they must make a buying decision today so they don't miss out on an opportunity that is available only at your health club or only today. An example of this is a first-visit incentive: "If you enroll on your first visit, you get X, and I am sure you don't want to miss out on getting X, do you?" Asking questions that are designed to elicit a no answer can also benefit your presentation. When you ask a question where you want a no answer, shake your head no very inconspicuously, and the prospect will mirror your actions by shaking his or her head and responding with a no answer. It is difficult (unnatural) for someone to say yes when he or she is shaking his or her head no. Use this same technique if you want the prospect to answer your question with a yes; move your head up and down to encourage a yes response. If you don't think this technique really works, try it on your family and friends for fun, and you'll be amazed.

- Frustration: "Do you feel as if you are not achieving your goals because you feel you are unhealthy and unfit? Are you facing obstacles that seem overwhelming?" Show your prospects how a health-club membership will help them achieve their goals because of the renewed energy and positive outlook they will experience if they are members of the club. When they work out, they will feel great.

- Worry: "Do you worry about your longevity because of poor lifestyle choices? Do you worry about diabetes, heart failure, stroke, and other preventable diseases?" Show prospects how a health-club membership will help them have control over their lives by being fit and healthy.

- Discontent: "Do you feel envy for other people who are living healthy lifestyles or enjoying more active lifestyles?" Show prospects how a health-club membership will give them access to a healthier lifestyle. Introduce them to members who fit the same profile of health-conscious consumers, and show them that they can also socialize with health-and-fitness-conscious people for motivation and inspiration.

- Anger: "Does your anger due to failure in this aspect of your life agitate you and keep you from doing the things you are supposed to do? Do you feel grumpy, bad tempered, and easily annoyed because there is no stability in your life?" Becoming a member of the club can add stability to their lives because they will have a sense of belonging and have something exciting to look forward to everyday, such as going to the gym and socializing with people who have the same interests.

- Regret: "Do you ever feel regret when thinking of past mistakes, failures, defeats, and lost opportunities as they pertain to your health?" Let prospects know that if they do not buy a health-club membership today, it will be something they might have to add to their growing list of regrets.

- Embarrassment: "Do you feel embarrassed about your present fitness situation?" Show prospects how a health-club membership can save them from the embarrassment they are feeling right now by making them imagine their ideal bodies while they are with other healthy and fit new friends, hanging out and so on.
- Hopelessness: "Do you feel you are drifting aimlessly in life without the hope it can get better?" A health-club membership will give prospects new direction and will open up new opportunities for them.
- Sadness: "Do you feel unsatisfied with your life? Are you feeling miserable, depressed, and gloomy because of your weight?" A health-club membership will help prospects meet new people and build new relationships that will give new meaning to their lives.
- Guilt: "Do you feel guilty taking care of yourself?" Tell prospects they can alleviate those guilty feelings with a health-club membership, because being healthy is the best thing they can do for their families. Ask the prospect this question: "If a dollar a day can add five to ten years to your life, is it worth it to you?"

Compose some questions that bring up positive emotions, like the following:

- Achievement: "How does joining the club today contribute to the goals you set for yourself? How would it feel to be the first among your relatives or friends to actually achieve your weight goals? Every little step you make to improve your life is considered an achievement."

- Pride: "Wouldn't you be proud to be a member of this club?" Prospects can take pride in being part of a group of health-and-fitness-conscious people. They can feel proud they are taking good care of their bodies. "How proud of yourself will you be when you achieve your fitness goals?"

- Security: Design questions to elicit this emotion, for example, how does joining today offer your prospect a sense of security? Security is a blanket emotion that includes money, love, acceptance, power, and control. Let prospects know that living a healthy lifestyle will make them happier and more productive people, which will help them attract and build new relationships, become more efficient at work or when running their own businesses, discover new opportunities, and so on.

- Self-improvement: "Are you goal oriented? Is striving to be better important to you? When you are part of a club or organization, you become more confident because you see results." Find out how joining today will appeal to the prospect's sense of self-improvement.

- Status: "What do you think your coworkers will say when they see the new you?" Discover how a health-club membership will contribute to the status of your prospect. Does being a member of a health club make him or her feel important? By looking successful in the eyes of their peers, prospects will feel more significant.

- Style: "Are you ready to wear skinny jeans again?" How does a health-club membership fit, enhance, or manifest your prospect's sense of style? Let your prospect know that leading a healthy lifestyle will never go out of style.

- Conformity: "Are you ready to make a commitment to a healthy lifestyle?" (This question can also be used as a test-closing question which I'll cover later in this chapter.) How does a health-club membership offer the comfort and safety of the crowd? Let your prospects know that an extraordinary life requires them to be healthy and fit, and if they want to lead successful lives, they must conform to a healthy lifestyle.

- Ambition: "Did you know that corporations look at applicants' lifestyles when choosing who best fits the company's long-term goals?" Ask how a health-club membership will help the prospect get more out of life and get ahead.

- Power: "Picture yourself strong and fit in a power pose; can't you see yourself getting that new job, getting that beautiful girl, and winning in life?" In what ways does a health-club membership offer prospects more power or control over their lives? A health-club membership will give prospects a new perspective on life, satisfying all six core emotional needs (certainty, variety, significance, love and connection, growth, and contribution), while giving them the power to feel in control of their lives.

- Love: "If you were at your ideal weight and in peak shape, would you feel better about your relationships? Wouldn't you feel you had more energy to give more in your relationships? Would you feel more attractive to the opposite sex? Would you have more confidence to go after the person of your dreams?" In what ways does a health-club membership allow prospects to feel love and connection? A health club provides a safe platform for members to connect with new friends, build long-term relationships, and take risks.

By this time, you should already have the pertinent information you need to get the prospect to make the buying decision today. The prospect must have enough want and must have justification as to why he or she must buy now, and if he or she doesn't, you did a poor job on the interview and tour. You must learn to pick up on body language that can tell you when the prospect is ready to buy: facial expressions, posture, vocabulary, and actions. For example, if prospects' facial muscles are tight (not in an irritated way but because they are deep in thought) and if they are scratching their chins, they are giving the decision great thought. The more relaxed the prospect is, the closer to buying he or she is. If you put something like a brochure or contract in front of the prospect and they start touching it or asking questions about it, they are more likely to say yes. If prospects are smiling a little more often than they had in the beginning of the presentation, their attitudes are friendly and they are aligning with you they are probably ready to buy. If prospects are excited, their eyes will open a little wider, and their pupils will slightly dilate. If prospects are leaning forward, they are listening more intently; they are really attentive and interested in what you have to say and will ask questions. All of these "tells" are signaling that the prospect is ready to buy. You must watch for these signs and take appropriate action: lock up the relationship, and close the sale.

Closing

Always begin your presentation by knowing where you stand. Is the prospect hot or cold? Take his or her temperature by asking test-closing questions. Test-closing questions are opinion-asking questions; opinion questions are not decision questions. Start with a question like, "In your opinion, do you feel enrolling today would be the best first step toward reclaiming your life?" By test closing, you avoid overselling, like selling the membership during the interview and tour, and then buying it back because you don't know when to shut up or you go for the close too fast ("buying it back" is a sales term for not knowing when to shut up, which can cost you a sale and therefore a missed opportunity to earn a commission).

Here are a couple of test-closing questions:

1. How long have you been considering enrolling in a health-club membership? You are not asking the prospect if they want to join today; you are just digging deeper to see if they have already formed an opinion about enrolling anytime in their life.
2. If you can live longer by spending a dollar a day, is it worth it to you?
3. I know you are concerned about _____, but wouldn't it be worth _____ to get _____ (some benefit)? (The benefit must be strong enough to provide leverage to move them away from their fears.)

Test closing allows you to shed light on the no's, for example, no I don't want to buy, no I'm not ready now, and overcome them before they are verbalized. Do not hide from no's; everyone will get them, so welcome them. This far into the presentation, the no's are easy because they're "not yets," and you're not asking prospects to buy now; you're just finding out what they're thinking at this point. Don't use the shotgun approach and try to attack every objection head on. Use test-closing questions to get those objections out so you can take them out like a fine-tuned sniper—one at a time.

If you're always test closing, you'll know what kind of state of mind the prospect is in. Notice if you're moving him or her toward making a commitment or away from a commitment. If he or she is moving in the wrong direction, make a change in your presentation. Never ask the customer to buy until you are positive he or she is ready. You accomplish this, of course, through test closing. This helps you and your ego as well, because this way, you never feel rejected and are always comfortable and confident throughout the presentation.

Here are some other test-closing questions:

1. If you were to go ahead with a health-club membership, when would you want it to start? This question is designed to see if the prospect has formed an option on joining today or is still procrastinating.
2. If we were able to overcome _____, would you be ready to move forward today?
3. Does this membership package sound like it will serve your needs?

When you feel the prospect is ready to join, go for the close (assume the close means the prospect has already given you the go ahead with the membership whether verbally or nonverbally) by going right into the paperwork. I prefer "go for the close," because I never "assume" anything but it is an industry term, so I would be remiss if I didn't teach it to you.

Even though all of the sales process should have been done during the interview and tour, you may still get some pushback during the paperwork. Do not panic; you should only panic if you have failed to lay the groundwork. Objections are just a cry for more information; celebrate objections. When prospects raise objections, it means they're interested but need more information. Objections at this point are no problem because now you know what is stopping the prospect from making the commitment. Now you know what direction to go in and where to build more value or eliminate pain.

Most objections are questions in disguise, begging to be answered. When you uncover an objection that you have no control over as a salesperson—décor, equipment, programs—find a way to brag about it or overcome it. The best example of this is a time I met this old club guy who I heard was a great salesman, so I asked whether he would mind taking me on a tour of his club. I must preface this story by saying the club we were in was a dump. As he was taking me on a tour, I commented that the carpet was full of holes, the vinyl on the equipment was worn out, and the paint was chipping off the wall. This didn't deter him in the least. He responded,

> "This carpet is in rough shape because our happy members wear it out yearly just to secure spots in the front of our world-class aerobic classes. This vinyl—our members love this equipment so much and are losing so much weight that we can't change the vinyl fast enough. And look at these walls; the members have such a great time here socializing that the crowds rub the paint off the walls. But you know what? We don't care, because we love our members, and they love us."

The best thing of all was when he was speaking, he came across as sincere and caring. He knew the power of body language, enthusiasm transfer, and mirroring. He was using his hands with enthusiasm and shaking his head yes the entire time. I was sold!

Here are some other ways of handling objections. Always remember questions are a salesperson's best friend, so learn to use them to overcome objections. Never argue or go against what the prospect says or feels. Always align with them. Always answer the questions presented to you. Some salespeople follow the school of thought that you can ignore questions and they will disappear, but I believe all questions should be addressed now, so there is no buyer's remorse tomorrow. Turn an objection into a question. For example, when they say, "It's too expensive," ask them, "Can you tell me the reason why you think it costs too much?" Questions are powerful; you can always turn an objection into a question. Ask questions that make prospects focus on benefits as opposed to their concerns.

Here are a few examples of how to turn objections into questions. Use any of the four objections (time, money, spouse, or think about it) or insert your own:

- In spite of _____, isn't it possible you can still get enormous value from our membership? Don't you think you can still achieve _____ (the prospect's benefits) from our membership?
- How can we get _____ (benefit) without you having to continue to suffer?
- How do we do _____ so you still can benefit from joining today?
- Wouldn't it be great if we could find a way to accomplish _____?
- Do you no longer worry about _____?
- Why would _____ even be an issue since you've been telling me how desperate you are for a change?

Turn the objection back to the prospect. If they say, "I don't have the money," then respond, "That's exactly why you must buy it today. You will save an enormous amount of money if you enroll today, and as everyone knows, money saved is money earned."

Overpower objections like "I need to think about it" by piling on more and more reasons why they must buy now because they have already been thinking about it for years.

Some of the examples of questions given in this book are never going to feel comfortable to you. These questions are just examples. You must design your own questions that fit your social style so you can ask them with conviction. Don't read these examples and say "I could never say that." Ask yourself, "How can I ask that question in a way that suits my style, or what would be a better question for me to ask than that?"

Move to make an objection a final objection—for example, "If we can agree on *X*, are you ready to move forward to the paperwork?"

After overcoming an objection and getting positive feedback from the prospect, go for the close. Congratulate the prospect on making a wise decision, and shake hands with him or her. Take out the agreement (contract), and start filling it out.

Go for the close by asking, "How would you like to take care of your membership today: Visa or MasterCard?" Too many options are confusing—avoid brain overload! Limit the options to two choices. Less is more. Lots of options confuse people, and they will opt not to choose at all. Too many choices tax the lazy brain. Your brain is always looking for ways to conserve energy because it functions on only twelve watts of power. That is why it is difficult for people to make a choice or decision if there are too many options. Reduce the possibilities of confusion by limiting the choices. Make it easy to buy today.

Don't say another word when you ask your closing question; remember, a closing question is a make-a-decision question. If you wait for the customer to answer, he or she will, and it will probably be one of your choices, for example, Visa or MasterCard; if you speak first, you start the entire sales process over. Sometimes, the silence will seem to last an hour. Just be patient, and wait; you'll be very happy you did. Whoever speaks first will lose. The only acceptable pressure in a professional-sales presentation is silence; use it. Remember, by losing (speaking first), the prospect wins because now they will stop procrastinating and start a new way of life today.

After finalizing the paperwork, you must create a compelling future for the new member. Have the new member explain to you how he or she plans on changing his or her life since he or she has now joined the club. Ask him or her, "A year from now, what do you think will stand out as being one of the best things that came from you enrolling today?" Now the new member will be able to justify the purchase when talking to his or her peers, spouse, kids, and so on so he or she doesn't get pushback about the purchase.

Always give a gift at the close to induce reciprocation. It makes someone feel committed. Give a gym bag, a sweat towel, a free-tanning-for-a-week certificate, or anything of value at the signing of the contract. After giving new members (tangible) gifts, do you think they will ever back out? Unlikely. It's called the rule of reciprocity; you give them a bag, and they give you their loyalty.

Convert this new relationship into future business. Ask new members before they leave whether they would fill out a buddy-referral sheet (this is part of the free download). If you feel it is necessary, offer them something in return. Get as much info on the referrals as possible. Even on presentations you don't close, get referrals. Say to the prospects who chose not to join, "I understand you feel this may not be the right fit for you at this time. Do you know of someone who could benefit from our membership?" Sometimes, prospects will be glad to give you someone else because they'll feel they are no longer in your cross hairs: this theory is called see a shark, stab your dive buddy.

If you haven't already, go get the free download at healthclub-marketingmmc.com. Between what you have learned here today and what you'll receive in the free download, you will be able to confidently sell any health-and-fitness product or service to any prospect in the world. If you have comments, please feel free to e-mail me at chuck@chuckthompson.guru (not dot com). Good luck, and now, let's get back to New York.

CHAPTER 4

SELLING CLUB MEMBERSHIPS BY THE THOUSANDS

I had the George Washington Bridge in sight—I was on my way to the Big Apple, and man, was I excited. Most people would be thrilled about going to New York for the shows, restaurants, and nightlife, but not me; I was happy to get back in the action of selling memberships and just wanted to go straight to work. I have worked for most of my life and am the kind of guy who needs to be making things happen, not sitting by a phone, waiting for a call. New York meant only one thing to me—success: I was determined to make it there because I knew I could make it anywhere (as the song New York New York goes, slightly revised). I was ready to prove myself anywhere, so why not in the Big Apple? I had no plans on seeing the sights; I just wanted to know the location of the club where I'd be working and the hotel where I would be staying so I could get checked in and start doing some recon.

I would call the promoter's office every night and give his secretary an update on my whereabouts and estimated time of arrival. The night before I was to arrive in the Big Apple, the secretary told me there had been a change of plans. I would now be stopping just short of New York in Secaucus, New Jersey, to set up one of the three health clubs in the chain. These clubs carried an NFL player's name but were operated by his partner(s). The other two clubs were in Long Island, New York, which is where I originally thought I would be going.

The promoter's secretary informed me they had already taken care of my reservations and I was to check in at a local motel. Having my motel reservations handled by someone else like this was a first for me, but I was so excited about the opportunity, I didn't even think to make any requests; besides, the promoter and I had met at one of the nicest hotels in Dallas, and both of the promoters were very well dressed, so I assumed I would be receiving at least middle-class accommodations. Boy, was I stupid to assume. The promoter's secretary neglected to tell me the motel reserved for me was on skid row (pre–Google Maps). I arrived at this motel, and there were drug dealers, pimps, and prostitutes everywhere. The place was a dump with century-old sheets, nasty carpets, and paper-thin walls; I was furious, to say the least. I called the office and gave the secretary a piece of my mind. I was used to motels (as opposed to hotels) at that point in my life because I was still struggling financially, but these were the worst accommodations you could imagine. They assured me it was only for a few nights, because all of the hotels in the area were fully booked, and I would be moved as quickly as possible. Since I wasn't rolling in money and had spent most of what I had partying in Dallas and on the expenses of getting to New Jersey, I had no choice but to accept it. So, I made the best of things, called my flight-attendant friend, and asked her to jump on a plane and fly out to spend a few days with me while I set up the promotion.

The next morning, I woke up and immediately went to the club to check it out. It was very nice but a pain in the behind to get to. It was facing a main thoroughfare with huge concrete dividers, so if you missed your turn, you were forced to drive five miles out of the way to find a turnaround. There was no one in the club when I got there that morning, which wasn't too unusual, since most clubs have a morning crowd and an evening crowd, and just do the best they can to get some people in from 9:00 a.m. until 4:00 p.m. I loved the property because the club was completely modern. Secaucus, New Jersey, back in the mid-1980s was literally meadowlands and industrial parks. The area where they had put this club was definitely the nicest part of Secaucus, but there were very few homes nearby, and that concerned me a little. I knew now why I was in New Jersey, and the promoter sent his girlfriend to New York: this club needed a hustler, not a Barbie doll.

The promoter wanted me to put out fifty lead boxes to start generating some cash. The promoter was fronting the initial cash for the hotels where his salespeople were staying, and he needed to raise some cash quickly to pay for the newspaper and radio ads to recoup his hotel costs and give him some working capital. I also realized that was why I was in the cheapest motel in the entire state of New Jersey: the promoter needed to raise some money before he could afford to put me in a decent hotel.

Lead boxes are registration boxes you see in stores, usually near the cash registers or on the checkout counters. They have big letters reading that if you register, you'll win something for free. In the health-club business, the top prize would normally be a free trip to the Bahamas or somewhere tropical, or a free one-year health-club membership. The vast majority (99.9 percent) of the people who entered to win a trip to the Bahamas won a free two-week pass to the health club. It was an easy way to generate leads and get people through the door and excited about the club's services. Sometime during the two-week trial, or preferably during the first visit or workout, the two-week-pass holder would be given the opportunity to enroll, with some kind of first-visit discount or incentive. In most cases, it was an offer to trade in his or her two-week-pass for a discounted membership rate or for no initiation fee. It sounds too easy, but lead boxes worked well.

It was also fairly easy to get businesses to put the lead boxes in their stores because health clubs always offered some kind of incentive in the form of memberships to the owners or managers for displaying the boxes in their store. But most membership coordinators were too lazy to put them out, much less check the boxes at least three times a week and invest the time and energy to work the leads generated turning the leads into new memberships. The boxes need to be checked a minimum of three times a week, or they might become full and start to look messy, thus pissing off the management of the business where the box was placed; even worse, some guy from another club might steal your leads. It sounds insane, but a lot of salespeople got their leads stolen, so I always seeded my boxes with a fake name and my telephone number so no one would know it was me. Then if someone ever called me, I'd go to the appointment and give the salesperson a personal lesson on ethics. But, I was fortunate because my reputation always preceded me in those early days in Nashville, and I didn't have to deal with that BS. I made it a point to take care of all the managers where I had put the boxes when they came in the club. I'd make sure they met all the hot girls; I gave them tanning passes, free personal-training sessions, and so on. Remember one hand washes the other; always take care of those who take care of you. You're building a brand, whether you know it or not.

I was a good soldier and did what the promoter asked of me and more. I think I put out almost one hundred lead boxes all over town, and since lead boxes were new to that area, I didn't have to worry about other salespeople stealing my leads. The home office would send supplies to the Jersey club for all three clubs, but the other salespeople were too lazy or too full of themselves to put out their shares of the lead boxes, so I put out every one that was left behind for my club. I didn't care about being seen as a big shot; we were all poor, and all I cared about was rockin' this club. I would collect the leads every day and call the registrants and inform them they had won a free two-week pass to the club. The prospect was always overjoyed because everyone loves to win, and everyone loves getting free stuff. But the main reason prospects came in to take advantage of the free offer was because it held real emotional and monetary value. They wouldn't have come in for a one-day pass or for an open house designed to sell them something; in their minds, they were winners coming in to pick up their prize. Within a week or so, I had sold a ton of memberships and sent the cash straight to the promoter's office in Michigan. I wish I could say it was my sales acumen that was responsible for the success of this promotion. Yes, I did all of the legwork to get prospects in the door, but the club was so nice and the price was so cheap, everyone and his or her brother bought a membership.

I love being busy, and it was busy. It wasn't long until the ads were out in the newspapers, and the place was jumping. I was sending overnight envelopes full of checks and cash through FedEx daily. The promoter wanted the cash immediately, so the home office had us send it in every day. I was collecting money from twenty, forty, and even sixty people at one time; it was crazy busy. Soon, I had to hire a couple of local girls to give group tours and bring the guests to me in the nursery room, where I would close the sale. Then, I had another girl taking cash, checks, and credit cards, sitting behind a folding table. I had to set up the operation in the nursery because there were so many guests, and most of them came in between 4:00 p.m. and 8:00 p.m., which created traffic jams at the front desk, because the existing members were checking in at the same time. Moving to the nursery alleviated the traffic problem and also hid the crowds of new members from the original members. Overcrowding is always a major concern for club owners, but in reality, it is very unlikely that a club will become overcrowded when you take everything into consideration: hours of operation; days per week each member works out; percentage of members who come to the club only once a month, twice a month, or three times a year; and so on. Nonetheless, you don't want to raise the issue among members, so it is best to avoid backing up the front counter.

One of the selling points of this company was that the promotion company brought in their own staff to sell all the memberships so the club owner wouldn't have to rely on his "inferior" sales staff. They would hype up the salespeople as though they were the Joe Girard (listed in the *Guinness Book of World Records* as the greatest salesperson) of the health-club industry. In reality, these salespeople didn't know anything about sales and knew even less about the health-club industry, but they were good-looking, and sometimes all it takes is good looks to get your foot in the door. This is another psychological phenomenon: people with perfectly shaped faces are trusted at first, more than people who are not as universally considered beautiful. This is based on familiarity; the one- to one-point-five ratio face is the most common shape, and people relate more to what they are accustomed to. The fact of the matter is the promoter's staff was in the club only to make sure the money was collected and sent back to the promoter. The promotion company's managers actually hired temporarily local people to do the sales (order taking). I love the craft of professional sales, and later when I became aware of this misrepresentation it did not sit well with me at all.

The Secaucus club did very well and far exceeded the promoter's expectations. I heard the final totals for those three clubs was around $1.8 million in cash collected in just sixty days. This was fantastic for the nine thousand new members and the promoter, but the owners took it in the shorts because they didn't make near as much money as they thought they would have. Don't get me wrong; at the time, I was ecstatic with the results because I was learning and had just helped thousands of people take their first step toward healthier lifestyles. I also earned a decent commission for my efforts.

Asking me to sell memberships one by one was like hiring Van Gogh to paint your car. I wanted to be out selling promotions to club owners. You could have taught a monkey to do the job I was doing. The promoter knew this too; I was his thoroughbred, and it was stupid to keep me in the barn. He needed to turn me lose and let me do what he hired me to do: lock up business relationships. I could see the future of the health-club business beginning to outgrow its customer base, and I knew there would be a wider market for this type of promotion in the coming years. Everyone wanted in on the action of owning a health club, and there were gyms and health clubs being built on every corner. There was absolutely no way all of these clubs were going to survive without effective marketing; it just wasn't mathematically possible. You would think some of these owners with their postgraduate degrees (doctors and lawyers) would have known this, but they still kept building.

Finally, I had found the platform I needed to sell health and fitness to thousands of people. I wanted to sell promotions to health-club owners so I could increase membership sales on a mass scale. The promoter and his partner knew this about me, and as soon as the promotion in New York and New Jersey ended, the promoter sent me to his partner's home in Marietta, Georgia, for training on how to sell the promotion to club owners. I thought the idea of me being trained on sales by the partner a bit comical though, since the partner had brought the promoter in as a partner in his business because he couldn't close the big deal with the three clubs in New York and New Jersey in the first place. By the end of the promotion, the brought-in partner who I have been referring to as the promoter actually took over the whole company and was giving the original (Georgia) owner the leftover crumbs. It was the old adage in real life: "A man with money meets a man with experience; the man with the experience walks away with the money, and the man with the money walks away with experience." But I had taught myself to be open-minded because I could learn something from everyone's successes and failures, just as I had over the course of my career. So, I eagerly headed back down south to Marietta, Georgia, which is a beautiful upscale suburb just north of Atlanta.

In Georgia, I was looking forward to my conversations with the partner. We had met only once in Texas, and even then, I had appreciated his enthusiasm. It didn't hurt that he had also been impressed with my energy and the depth of knowledge I had about the industry, so we had a mutual respect and admiration. He was a short, well-dressed, and well-spoken man who had bought the company from another guy who had previously worked with his new partner. Long story short, we knew a lot of the same industry people, and he was able to give me a close, personal look at the genealogy of the promotion business. I could tell right away in our meeting in Dallas that he wasn't an alpha male, and I kind of felt sorry for him because I could see the promoter was definitely in charge, even though it was supposed to be this guy's company. I had spent the past five years learning how to read people, and this story wasn't going to end well for him, but it was none of my business.

I stayed at his home in Georgia for a few days and visited a chain of clubs he had run the promotion for to get the owner's perspective, and just as I thought, the owner was glad he had run the promotion, because he had needed the cash. He also wished it had been structured differently, because he had no additional revenue for the long-term financial health of his club. He said they had sold the memberships for $99 a year, and it went gangbusters. I said of course it did. A health-club membership in the mid-1980s averaged $600 a year. Some clubs' prices were as high as $1,500 per year. Every person mildly interested in fitness would join for $99 per year; it was a no-brainer. I thanked the gentleman for his time and gave him one of my manuals. I told him that since he now had a ton of members who had gotten such a great deal, he should implement an aggressive referral program to get some full-paying members in the club to offset the others, and I was confident that if he trained his staff with my system, he would have a great year. The law of reciprocity always works, and since he gave the members such a great value, the majority would want to reciprocate.

I am always looking for ways to turn lemons into lemonade. When I'm faced with challenges, I ask myself, how can I make this work? Success is simple mathematics; just having that many bodies in the club should bring in a ton of buddies and profit-center revenue. The worst part of the promotion wasn't even that there was no up-sale but that the promotion focused only on the health-and-fitness-conscious consumer and didn't penetrate any other segment. In short, the club cannibalized its own membership and then sold ninety-nine-dollar memberships to prospects who would have easily paid rack rates. In essence, they literally gave the club away.

The amazing thing about the club owner in Atlanta was that at the end of our conversation, he said he had a lot of friends in the industry, and he had told everyone about the promotion and how well it had done in his clubs. This is one of the earliest problems that plagued the industry: club owners as well as their staff wanted to share their experiences with other industry people. Owners and staff get so blinded by the traffic and cash that is flowing, they fail to share the whole story, which makes sense since they don't know the whole story—they only know about 10 percent of the promotion. They shared everything they knew, like the price-point, the promotional pieces (letters and newspaper ads), and the forms they received. What they failed to tell the other clubs is the promotion company did 90 percent of everything behind the scenes, and the only thing the club received was the 10 percent of the knowledge necessary to successfully take the orders, and that 10 percent of knowledge can only help them capture consumers who were already customers.

I had been immersed in the health-club industry for about six years at that time and had just run a promotion for the company, which meant I was far more involved and informed than any owner or staff member, yet I was still 80 percent in the dark, and the promoters were teaching me everything they could as fast as they could so I could sell club owners on the promotion. So, being told by the club owner he had shared all the information with his friends in the industry just baffled me. Basically, what he really did was give them just enough rope to hang themselves—bankrupt their business.

I went back to the partner's house, and we made some cold calls for a few days to set up some appointments. I had gotten in the habit of making ten appointments minimum per day when I was selling memberships face-to-face in the clubs, but now, I was going to be driving all over the country, so I decided I would set up ten appointments per week (two a day, five days per week), and then the following week, I would go back for my follow-ups and fill in the rest of the time doing drop-ins and making new appointments for the next week. These promoters who I was working for didn't know what to think of my detailed planning and aggressive approach to traveling state to state, because they had never worked like this. They had been living on a few sales per year and making as much money as they could off each deal. But both of them were older than I was and had already established themselves financially. I only had my commissions from the Jersey club to live on, and I was going to be responsible for all of my own travel expenses, so I needed a workable system.

It was easy making appointments because I designed a killer presentation. I had learned a long time earlier the most important thing to lead with is what's in it for the prospect. If you don't capture the prospect's attention in the first ten seconds, you've lost him or her forever, so you must always start off with what is in it for him or her. I would call an owner and tell him or her the promotion company puts up all of the money and provided the sales staff. This is called risk reversal for the prospect while selling the results of your company's product. Club owners ate it up. Most clubs were starting to feel pressured from so many new clubs popping up; they were willing to listen to anything new. In 1987, very few people had heard of promotion companies, and if no other club within their area had run a promotion like this, the whole concept was completely foreign to them. Within a few days, I had my presentation down and had already made my ten appointments, so I was eager to get on the road.

There were four things I loved when I was younger. Here they are in order: women, learning, music, and traveling. Now, all four were a part of my daily life. I was ready to conquer the world. My first few appointments were pretty sloppy. I still didn't know the product, and my delivery was awkward, but I got better with each presentation. The promoters told me very little other than I was selling money, but club owners needed much more than mere money; they needed a sustainable model. Most owners saw the promotion for what it really was—a fire-sale. The clubs that had run the promotion and reached the big numbers only did so because no one in the marketplace had ever seen anything so radical. But once they ran it, most clubs were in more trouble than they were before the promotion. I realized I was having a hard time selling the program because I didn't believe in it either.

One of my biggest challenges in selling the promotion was its perception as a fire-sale or a Hail Mary. The promotion itself was a tough sell because it just sounded too cheap. An owner had to really be desperate to do it because there was no possibility for residual income. I felt like a priest coming to read the clubs' last rites.

After a few weeks, I sold my first promotion, and the promoter was thrilled. From that day on, I spent every dime of my commissions driving east to west and north to south, covering the entire United States. It takes a special kind of person to live on the road, but I loved traveling, seeing all types of clubs, learning different marketing strategies, and building new relationships (both business and personal) in every state. I was fortunate I was still a bachelor, because a marriage and kids could have never afforded me the freedom to literally drift from town to town. Living in hotels and sometimes in my car would have never sat well with raising a family, and the fun I was having being single made me feel like a rock star. This lifestyle was allowing me to live a life all boys dream of. Some kids grow up wanting to go pro so they can get the money and women, some want to become rock stars so they can get the money and women, and some want to become movie stars so they can get the money and women. I was the luckiest man on earth because even though I didn't have the money, I always had the women; I knew I was born to do this.

The company had about four independent salespeople out selling promotions, and one month, the promoter came up with a sales contest. The person who sold the most promotions the following month would win a new (leased) Mercedes Benz. The competition wasn't even close; I blew everyone out of the water and flew back to Michigan to pick up my new car. I was out in California at the time, so I took my T-bird to my grandmother's house and left it in her garage. My first Mercedes was a 1987 (if I remember correctly) champagne-gold 190E. It was beautiful, and man, it handled great. The only challenge was it was too small for me. I'm six feet four, and at the time, I weighed 220 pounds, so I almost had to sit in the back seat when I drove. But I didn't care; it was a Benz. I drove that car into the ground until I finally totaled it in an accident in Sacramento, California.

I was successfully selling the promotion because a lot of clubs were so desperate for cash, and one thing I was confident about was this promotion brought in some serious cash. I worked with clubs from California to Massachusetts and from Minnesota to Louisiana. The promoter would sometimes come out to spend a day or two with me, especially when I was working out a deal with a larger chain or a club with big potential. The promoter loved selling with me because I knew when to speak and when to shut up. The promoter resembled Richard Gere, and people really liked him and believed whatever he said, largely because of his looks and appearance, which made closing deals a lot easier for him. A couple of times when we were on the road together, he had call girls come to his room or picked up prostitutes off the street. I am not a choirboy by any stretch of the imagination, but this guy preferred prostitutes over the beautiful women we met in nightclubs. One night, we were having a drink in Chicago, on Rush Street, and we saw these girls dressed as hookers standing on a corner. They were really fine, and it was driving him crazy. He said, "Let's go talk to them." We walked over near them, and he looked around, checking out the situation to see whether there were any cops around. Once he thought the coast was clear, he moved in to proposition them, and just as he got within a few feet of the girls, a camera crew and a security team popped out of nowhere. The film crew scared the crap out of the promoter. Those girls were actresses making a movie! I laughed until I almost pissed myself. Later I asked him, "What the hell is wrong with you? You can get the hottest women in the world, but you prefer working girls." I know this all sounds a little *Pretty Woman*-ish, but this took place two or three years before the release of that movie. Who knows? Maybe someone in the movie business met this guy too. It's funny; out of all the time I spent with the promoter that is the one thing I remember most—that and, of course, the Benz.

Back in the 1980s, the health-club business was the perfect business for guys who loved women and variety. I know this behavior is far from being politically correct today, and now is not tolerated in business, but the 1980s were different. Guys and even some gals got into the business because of the lifestyle. We were all young, fit, good-looking, and ambitious. This is why the promoter's love for working women was so mind-boggling because guys like us could walk in any health club around the country and leave with a beautiful hot date within an hour or so.

But my association with that promoter and his company was coming to an end because my heart just wasn't in it, and our values were polar opposites. I had a major problem with selling something I knew wasn't a win-win, and this wasn't by any stretch of the imagination. Even the people you think would be the winners (the new members) ended up losing because the clubs wouldn't have the funds to keep the maintenance and customer service up to par; most of the money generated by the promotion went to the promoter. Or even worse, the owners would sometimes take the money and run, leaving the membership without a club. As a teenager, I strayed from my core values and the lessons I had been taught about how to treat others and myself. When I moved from my hometown to Nashville, I made a conscious decision that I would never stray from those core values ever again. Even though this job selling promotions was good for me (I was learning, making great money, and having fun traveling) and great for my bosses, it did not serve the greater good; knowing that, I just couldn't sell their product with a clear conscience anymore.

Before resigning I made an attempt to get the promoter to make some necessary changes to the promotion. I called him and shared my concerns and even gave him some ways to improve the promotion. Always come up with a few solutions first before you approach your superiors with a problem. Even though I followed that rule, the promoter wouldn't budge. From his point of view, things were going fantastically, and he was not about to fix something that, in his mind, was not broken. It was obvious this company and I did not share the same values. He only cared about the money and couldn't have cared less about the longevity of the clubs he ran the promotion in. I wanted success more than almost anyone, but I was not willing to sell my soul to get it. I knew there was a better way, but it would mean the promoter would get far less of the revenue, and, of course, to him, that was not a viable option.

The way the promoter had structured his deals with health-club owners was unethical. The sales pitch was the promoter would put up the money for the promotion and split the net profits after the promotion company's expenses came out first. The promoter also neglected to tell the club owner which expenses were covered by the gross revenue. The short answer was—all of them. The sad truth was the promoter really only put up the money for the lead boxes (they used the same boxes over and over for every promotion), and the money generated from the boxes funded the launch of the promotion. The promoter exaggerated most of the other expenses as well, so by the time it was all said and done, the owner received the short end of the stick. After about a year, I became aware of the mechanics and dynamics of the promotion and realized my superiors and I were profiting off the hard work of club owners who were just trying to stay afloat. I wasn't about to gamble with my morals just to make a buck. I knew I could make great money doing just about anything, and I didn't need to mislead or take advantage of anyone to do it.

Previously, I had been courted by our competitor to come to work for them. The other promotion company had offered me a better commission structure and said they would listen to my ideas if I ever decided to represent them. This husband-and-wife team had gone up against me several times, forcing club owners to choose which company to partner with, and fortunately for me, I had won most of the time. So, they were extremely interested in my being on their side. Up until that point, I really hadn't considered their offers, because I knew they had stolen the program from the guys I was working for and were running the program exactly the same way—from a position of greed and not for the betterment of the industry.

The wife was rumored to be one of the promoter's ex-girlfriends whom he turned into a saleswoman. He had sent her out to run a promotion in Pennsylvania for a guy who was renting space from a tennis club and had put in a line of leased Nautilus equipment in the club. Basically, this guy was in a no-money-down situation. He was leasing the space as well as the equipment, which was a fantastic idea because he had absolutely no skin in the game. This is a perfect example of thinking outside the box, for all of you entrepreneurs out there. There is an old adage: "It takes money to make money." I added to that adage too: "It takes money to make money, but no one says it has to be your money." Always be looking for traditional as well as nontraditional resources to meet your needs. This other promoter really got lucky because the brand of the tennis club made his promotion go extremely well, which made him a ton of money. He then started dating the saleswoman, and they decided to start their own company. So, now they were competing against her ex-boyfriend.

The only reason I agreed to make the switch was because I was made to believe I was going to be allowed to make some changes in the overall promotion that would make it far better for the industry. At that point, I felt I needed to work for an established company because I was still somewhat ignorant of the mechanics of the entire promotion and knew nothing about what happened behind the scenes, including how the finances worked. It wasn't until much later that I unearthed the reality of it all.

Making the transition to the new promotion company was easy. I was selling exactly the same thing, just under a different name. As I stated earlier, I don't like going into a new job telling people how to run their business until I have proven myself, so I set out on the road to do exactly that. I started selling clubs on the promotion immediately, and things took off like a rocket. I once again was zigzagging across the country, visiting clubs and selling promotions.

When I was in Sacramento, I had met this sexy blonde who loved health and fitness and wanted to travel, so I picked her up, and we hit the road. She was really health-conscious, and eating on the road had been taking its toll on me, so having someone there to help me make healthier eating choices was a huge blessing. It also didn't hurt that she had a killer body. This girl had long blond hair and a Kardashian butt, which was a little too big for my taste, but she was cool as hell, and I knew we would have a blast touring the country together. Everyone always dreams of traveling, but when you do it for a living, it gets old really quick. It is a pain in the behind checking in and out of hotels, hauling your luggage in and out of the car, unpacking and packing every night, eating fast food, driving all night to get to your next meeting on time, and getting clothes dry-cleaned and laundered in a rush. Sometimes, you drive all night, and when you get to the hotel, you're informed they have lost your reservation and have given your room to another guest, and then to top it off, there is a convention in town, so you are forced to drive thirty miles out of your way to find an available room that you can afford, and on and on and on.

At that time in my life, I couldn't afford to fly and rent cars, because I paid all of my own expenses and was making only enough money to cover my travel and living expenses. This was also before Google, GPS, and Google Maps. So, I was mapping out driving routes at night and pulling over on the side of the road to get my bearings on where I was and where I needed to be. Later, when I could afford to fly and rent cars, traveling became even more of a pain in the behind because then I was dealing with the airlines canceling or delaying flights, lost luggage, airport traffic, rude staff, and lost car-rental reservations, sometimes cars were not in the stall where I was directed, so I had to get back on the shuttle to the airport to get another car and then take the shuttle back to the car lot to try to find the rental car all over again. It seemed like every day when I was on the road, there was at least one major challenge I had to deal with, but it was just a part of the job.

So, having the companionship of a lady who wanted to experience traveling and who was also health-conscious was definitely welcomed. We left California and headed east. I worked every city and state along the way. If I didn't have an appointment, I would stop, get a yellow-pages phone book, and start dropping in on clubs in the area. I never went a day, other than Sundays, without seeing a club. We followed this same routine all the way to Maine. As we passed through Massachusetts, I saw this beautiful maroon Lincoln Continental Mark VI. It was hot, and I needed another car because my Thunderbird had been driven to death. It had well over one hundred thousand miles, and I needed a bigger car because there were two of us now. I didn't say "a new car," because back then, I could never have afforded one, but I had decent credit and a down payment and was confident about the purchase, so I bought her. She was just like my woman: a beauty with junk in the trunk.

I traveled up and down the East Coast, and it was the health clubs' peak season, making it more difficult to sell promotions. Money started getting really tight, and after a couple of months, the promoter became even tighter when it came to an advance, so I started getting into survival mode. I told my friend it would be better if she went back to California because I was getting ready to hit some hard times and would be sleeping in my car for a while until I could get another club going. She offered to stay with me, but I just couldn't stomach the thought of being responsible for someone else being homeless. For me, it was no problem—I had lived in my car before—but I wasn't about to put that on another person, especially a girl. So, I convinced her to go back to Sacramento and then hit her with another bombshell: I couldn't afford to buy her a plane ticket, and unfortunately, I would have to put her on a Greyhound bus. She took it well but insisted on going to the grocery store first to get me some healthy food to keep in my car so at least I would eat healthy.

After going to the store, I took her to the bus station and headed out to the Massachusetts Turnpike to sleep at one of the oases (rest stops) along the highway so I wouldn't get in trouble with the police or get mugged. I found a great place and got settled in for the night. As I stated earlier, I am six feet four inches tall, and since it was a nice clear night, I decided to sleep with my feet hanging out the window, so I rolled my windows down for the night. Early in the morning, I started feeling these little needles sticking me in the face. I jumped up, wondering what the hell was going on, and I realized I was covered in bee and mosquito stings. I rolled out of the car, swatting and jumping around like somebody suffering from an epilepsy episode trying to get all of those bugs off of me. Later, I realized all of that damned fresh fruit my friend had bought and put in the back seat had drawn the bugs that were eating me alive. I laughed my butt off for years anytime I thought of that. Later, I thought maybe that was my karma for sending her 2,800 miles across the country on a Greyhound.

After a few weeks, I sold another club, and things got back to normal. I really wanted to implement my ideas, so within just a few months I insisted the owner hear me out. He suggested I come to Pennsylvania, where we would have a face-to-face chat. He also mentioned that everyone in the company wanted to meet me because I was a combination of a myth and a legend around the office. All of these clubs sold by Chuck Thompson were coming into the office of this promoter, but only the owner, his wife, and their VP had ever met me, so everyone wanted to see me in person. I was never much on socializing; I think it is mostly a waste of time. I've always been the guy who likes to work behind the scenes and make things happen. I was truly happy visiting clubs, reading, listening to my educational tapes, and learning from club owners about how they operated their businesses. You will never know or understand the depth of an education you'll get by working with clubs in every geographical area possible until you have done it yourself. No traditional institution of higher learning can ever come close to teaching what you learn by being there in person with your finger on the pulse.

When I got to Pennsylvania, all arms were open wide. The office girls were happy to see me, and the owner couldn't wait to show me all his material possessions, from his custom-built home to his shiny new Cadillac. His wife had already adjusted to the highbrow crowd and had a brand-new Mercedes 450SL. I couldn't help but be amused and disgusted at the same time: I was amused because they thought these material possessions would impress me, and disgusted because I was living in my car from time to time, selling promotions, so these two posers could feel significant and successful by flaunting their wealth. I had seen a lot of so-called rich people living in big homes like that one, mortgaged to the sky, desperately struggling to keep their image up and the lights on, while robbing from Peter and stealing from Paul just to keep living the lie that everything is going well with their finances, so I was not impressed in the least. In my travels, I have seen many businesspeople not make payroll or shortchange members on services they have paid for, all so they can live high on the hog. Don't get me wrong; I like nice homes and nice cars, but I'll never have them at the expense of others.

After dinner, the new promoter and I sat out on his lanai to have a discussion. He started pontificating about the promotions we had done and how much money he had made in the few short years he had been in the business. I could hear a real disconnect between his goals and the club owners' concerns and challenges. It was obvious his values were self-centered, because every time I brought up the concerns of the owners I had spoken with, he dismissed them as being irrelevant. I asked him numerous times how the clubs were going to grow if they sold these all-inclusive memberships for a ninety-nine-dollars a year, and he, in so many words, implied that it was their problem and not his. I was appalled by the conversation and knew it would be the last time I would be associated with him or his company. Things had been going really well for him and his family now that I was selling for him, and since I had left the other company, they had gone out of business, so he had no competition.

The next day, I received an early-morning call at my hotel asking me to come to the new promoter's office because he wanted to talk before I left. I agreed as a courtesy and packed my car and went straight over. He met me in the lobby of a small office building he had built from promotional dollars; it had a very sophisticated security system, which gave me pause. Back in the 1980s, no one had the elaborate security systems we have today. One, they were extremely expensive, and two, no one felt them to be that necessary. When I saw this, I thought, what the hell is this guy afraid of? He escorted me into the conference room and asked me to go through a presentation so he could record it. I knew exactly what was going on: he knew from last night's conversation I was on my way out, and he wanted to learn my presentation so he too wouldn't be out of business when I left.

This was par for the course with that guy. He thought he could copy and steal his way to the top. Just as he copied and stole the promotion, he thought if he had my presentation, he would be able to copy that as well. I knew where he got the idea of recording me, because in the past, when he asked, how I remembered so much about my presentations I had told him I recorded a lot of my presentations so I could study them in the car and at night in my hotel rooms. This was something I learned back when we would listen in on the presentations in the club in Nashville. I would go over the tapes (this was before smartphones) for hours, picking through the content with a fine-tooth comb. I was not only looking for what I was saying that was right but also looked for mistakes so I could eliminate them and not repeat them in the future. Other benefits of the recordings were the research and data I was compiling. Again, just as I learned about the four objections prospects raise in a membership presentation, I wanted to know club owners' core objections to the promotion. This is an education you'll never be able to comprehend unless it is you conducting the research.

One of the million things I have learned in my career is that a lot of people know what to do, but they don't always do what they know. For example, I put a free download on my company's website to teach anyone who wants to learn every step he or she needs to know to professionally sell health-club memberships, and yet most club managers and club salespeople still do not use this system the way it was designed. This simple step-by-step download could easily triple their income overnight, and it is absolutely free, yet they don't study and learn it. And when they do use it, they skip steps or even full sections. This system has been developed over thirty-five years and proven in over five hundred health clubs and over two hundred golf courses across America, and they still don't follow it correctly. I could have given the new promoter—or anyone else, for that matter—my presentation, but no one would ever be able to sell as I did. The biggest assets in my presentation are sincerity, empathy, honesty, and integrity—all values that are nonverbal and cannot be faked. So, as a parting gift and to give him something back for what I had learned while I represented his company, I recorded a couple of my presentations.

A year or so later, I received a call from a guy who introduced himself as an FBI agent. He went on to ask whether I knew my old boss, and of course I said I did. Then he asked me whether I was aware of his business practices and his associates, which I was not. I had only been to his office that one time, when I had made the decision to leave the company. The FBI agent proceeded to inform me that my ex-boss was under investigation for mail fraud and had connections to the mob. I informed the agent I was completely unaware of those issues. All I did was sell the promotion to clubs; I had no idea about the rest of the operations, nor did I ever meet any of his associates other than the VP—which was totally the truth. I heard later my ex-boss was sent to federal prison for mail fraud and tax evasion. Apparently, after I left he resorted to not only exaggerating the expenses of the promotions launched for clubs just like the original promoter but also claimed in his expense reports he was sending out more mail than he was. The club would get an expense sheet in the beginning of the promotion for X pieces of mail (even if the mail was not sent out), and all of those expenses, as well as the promoter's cut, would come out of the cash collected before the club owner saw a penny. I also heard some clubs never received a single dime of what was owed to them. The promoter's high-society lifestyle caught up with him and he chose a life of crime to keep up with the Joneses. He turned the whole promotion into a bigger scam than it already was, and I was so glad I got out when I did, because my conscience would have killed me had I known that one of my sales had been perverted in that way.

This is another thing that drives me nuts: when a salesperson for a promotional company goes out and convinces a club owner, he or she knows the business. Salespeople are taught how to sell the product, but that is all. No one I've ever met is as tenacious about learning as I am, and when I was a salesman, it consumed all my time just learning to sell the product well. I had no clue what went on behind the scenes; I just did what I was told and fulfilled my responsibilities, and that was to sell the promotion to club owners. I did not pretend to know the mechanics of the promotion, nor did I lie to owners and lead them to believe I did. When I presented the product, I let the owners know in no uncertain terms I was strictly the salesman and not the creator or operations person. I also made it very clear that once we finalized the paperwork, he or she (the new client) would be turned over to the office, and I was down the road to the next club. I let them know they could contact me via my beeper (I know, ha-ha, beeper) and I would respond ASAP, but the implementation of the promotion was in the hands of the office. People are all balls and no values if they can look someone in the eye and say they know how to run a promotion when they are only a sales representative. Club owners have their entire lives on the line and need competent help, not some con artist who is totally motivated by greed.

Quitting my job so abruptly definitely had its downside. The last thing I wanted to do was go back to selling health-club memberships one by one in another club. I also didn't want to simply manage a health club or find another company selling shady promotions. Consulting was an option, but I didn't want to keep making everyone else rich while I lived in my car. But after reviewing all of my options, I didn't know where else to turn but to consulting. I knew more about the health-club industry by this time than anyone else in the business. There were definitely industry guys who had been in the business a lot longer than I had been, but no one had the extensive hands-on experience in as many clubs across the United States as I did. In addition, by that time, my education had surpassed most graduate programs (had there been one) for professional membership sales. If I sat with an owner for just ten minutes, I could share enough of my knowledge to show him or her I would be an enormous asset to the business. I decided I would go back to a familiar place with tons of opportunity, so I set out for the Windy City—sweet home, Chicago.

I had a lot of relatives in Chicago. Both of my parents' siblings still lived there on the North Side, so I decided I would stay with my cousin for a few weeks until I could figure out my next step. Soon, I was running out of money because I had resigned so abruptly and hadn't had the foresight to save, so I decided to sell my Lincoln. Chicago has great public transportation, and I needed to pay rent because I was beginning to feel like a freeloader; I needed to be on my own, not living off other people. So, I gave my cousin a little money for back rent and went and rented an efficiency apartment near Wrigley Field. I was fortunate enough to meet a cute, petite southern blonde (natural brunette) from the hollers of Kentucky in a country bar on the northwest side of Chicago one night while I was staying with my cousin. She crashed at my new place and helped me forget about my financial woes and my conflicting feelings about the health-club industry, which I had loved for so many years and was now growing to hate. People make every decision in life either to avoid pain or to gain pleasure. Sometimes, you can have these two driving forces working at the same time, producing both pain and pleasure in response to the same thing. This is where I was in relation to the health-club industry. I knew getting a job would be easy, but I didn't want a job; I wanted to revolutionize the industry.

When I was eighteen, my father was shot and killed by a jealous woman, and the one thing he left me was his Yamaha acoustic guitar. My mother had scratched her name in the wood when they divorced so all his women would know she was the one who had bought the guitar for him. I carried it with me over the years, and it was like always having both of my parents there. I played the few chords my dad had taught me and picked up some more through the years, but I wanted to learn how to play well. My new girlfriend convinced me to go out to MI (Musicians Institute) in Hollywood, California, for a three-month summer course to get my head straight and just let things go and regroup. She said she would lend me the money and that when I came back, I could pay her back. So, I rented a van and headed out for California. It was so cool to be in school and be a student. I learned so much, but I soon realized playing guitar was a great hobby but not my passion. I was supposed to be studying scales, but all I could study was sales and marketing. Besides, I didn't need to learn to play guitar to be a rock star; I was already living the life of a rock star in the health-club business. I was supposed to be taking time off, but I was working harder studying than I would have been if I had a job; it was no vacation. As soon as the semester was over, I was back in Chicago and moved in with my girlfriend.

My parents instilled in me a work ethic that I could not suppress (and still can't to this day). I needed to go back to work. I had been thinking of some clubs I could call on in Chicago, and I remembered a chain of health clubs that desperately needed help but was too smart to sign on with the promotion that I had previously represented. I kept a log of all of the clubs I had presented the promotion to so I could stay in touch with the owners. The owners of that chain and I had hit it off well, and I knew they respected my honesty and integrity. I thought it wouldn't hurt to drop in on them and see whether they wanted to hire me as a consultant. We had had some great conversations in the past and agreed on the path their clubs should take to achieve their goals as a company. The husband and wife were just not sold on the fire-sale idea. By the time I met with them, it was at the end of my promotion days. I had lost all enthusiasm about the promotion as well, so I had halfheartedly presented the concept. I knew I was on my way out, and I was beginning to just go through the motions, which was a definite sign I was done with that type of promotion for good. I decided I would go by and see how they were doing and whether there might be a win-win for the both of us.

CHAPTER 5

MARKETING ESSENTIALS

Twelve Low- to No-Cost Marketing Ways to Increase Revenue Today

This new opportunity to manage four properties was with a chain of health clubs on the verge of bankruptcy. The two owners (both accountants) had bought the four clubs because they loved to play tennis, and one of the four clubs had tennis courts. They were a very nice couple who seldom got to play anymore because they were constantly plugging holes in a sinking ship (their business). They were very happy to see me, and within an hour, we were hammering out a compensation package where I would get a percentage of the gross revenue on all four clubs, as well as a salary, bonuses, and commissions on all personal sales. If nothing else, I was getting much better at negotiating my compensation package. The most important component of the compensation to me was the percentage of the overall company, which in my eyes was as good as being an owner without the overhead—in other words, I put nothing down and there was no downside for me. I had full operational control and felt I had finally arrived. Almost all the career industry guys and gals ultimately wanted to own their own health club, and here I was with a piece of the action and absolutely no skin in the game. Life was great again.

Those four health clubs were diamonds in the rough. Three of them were in great locations, and one was a dog in a downtown high-rise office building. The amenities were scattered over a couple of floors, and as I had learned earlier in my career, some downtown clubs can be challenging at best. I had also learned from my past experiences not to judge too quickly. So, for the first week, all I did was hang back and observe everything and everyone, from management down to the members. In most cases, when a business is failing, it is the owner's fault, and then the blame goes down the chain of command. The owner is responsible for getting great leadership (management), and the leadership is responsible for getting great soldiers (membership salespeople) on the team. In my mind, I was now an owner, and it was my responsibility to find and develop great leadership. So, one by one, I started chipping away at management. Some employees were relieved of their duties because they were either lazy or incompetent (and some were both). I didn't like doing it, but it had to be done. I believe if there is a cancerous cell, it must be removed, or it will inevitably cannibalize everything it touches. I retrained some people to finally do their jobs and do them well. I started with the troublemakers, and soon, everyone fell in line. I hired a ton of membership coordinators (salespeople) on draw salaries, kept the ones who could perform their duties well, and said good-bye to those who fell short. I stayed away from my previous criteria for membership coordinators (looks and gender) and relied 100 percent on membership-sales performance. I had a mission and a clear-cut goal to bring these health clubs out of desperation and propel them into jubilation.

I hired a sales force who loved to sell. You can teach most people how to lift weights properly or how to teach group classes, but you can't teach drive, heart, and determination. The people who already had these characteristics were the people I sought after to recruit. I made them sell me on why I should hire them. Since the clubs were in Chicago and Chicago suburbs, I had a much larger pool of applicants which afforded me the luxury of being able to pick and choose the right people for the job. Unfortunately, businesses located in areas with much smaller populations don't have this access to as many applicants and are often forced to take what they can get when it comes to employees.

Everywhere I went I gave out business cards; when I saw a good sales clerk, waiter, or anyone I thought was a go-getter. Within a few months, we had a first-class management team as well as a professional membership-sales team. I taught all of the workers in the clubs, from the janitor to the bookkeeper, how to sell within their own comfort levels and made them all feel they were important parts of the team. They were also rewarded financially and fairly for every sale they generated. I dug deep to unearth their personal goals, their likes, what motivated them, and then I coached them on how to make their dreams a reality. A key thing I learned was, you must hire people who love sales for sales positions, accountants for accounting positions, and attorneys for legal advice. I never ask my salespeople to do the bookkeeping, nor do I ask the bookkeeper for legal advice. I taught janitors and bookkeepers to hand out free passes to their friends, neighbors, relatives, and so on. When those people came into the club, it was the sales staff who sold the memberships, but both the salesperson and the person who generated the lead shared the commission.

Something that comes up a lot in my career is owners expecting their managers to be great marketers or salespeople. Each person has a specific skill set determined primarily by his or her passion. If the person you hire for marketing hates or despises sales, he or she will never be able to grow the business effectively. The person in charge of marketing must love sales and marketing; so if you can only afford to hire one person for management and sales, make salesmanship the qualifier.

Within a few short months, the clubs were out of the red and in the black. By that time, I was trying my hand at marketing campaigns and promotions, and I was knocking them out of the park.

I was not making the same mistakes as the promotion guys or the clubs they worked with by using a model that would eventually implode. I was being innovative, creative, and having fun. For me, this was what life was all about. Finally, I was actually fulfilling my need for contribution on a mass scale; I love contributing to the success of others. As I said before, I had a log of clubs whom I had presented the promotion to and also a list of the clubs I had sold the promotion to in the past, and I felt I owed them as much help as I could give them. I started offering my services free of charge to all clubs that wanted my help, which of course were most of them. I selected clubs located throughout the United States and nowhere near the four clubs I was currently representing, so there was absolutely no conflict of interest.

I was much more serious about my position and had curbed my extracurricular activities in the health clubs. My past experiences played a big role in my change, getting older and growing up was other contributed factors, but I was also in a great relationship with someone I really cared about, which is why I was able to completely focus on the task at hand-growing the company. I was so focused on the success of the company I didn't even realize how much I had changed. Actually, it was my girlfriend who pointed it out to me. It was as much subconscious as it was conscious.

I was going in early and working (only working) late. I was crunching numbers and planning the next day's membership-sales training every night. I was focused on daily goals and using a prepared schedule of tasks to accomplish them. I never let a day go by without inspecting what I expected. Accomplishing daily goals makes it easier to accomplish weekly goals, which in turn allows us to achieve and surpass our monthly goals. Question: How do you eat an elephant? Answer: one bite at a time. This is also referred to as chunking in the world of time management. When you have a big project, always break it down into small things so it doesn't get overwhelming.

I was getting more organized and started keeping even more thorough records on everything I did. I tracked marketing responses from the different media I was using to weed out the marketing efforts that weren't performing and kept the ones that worked best. I tracked closing percentages on all membership sales to isolate successful strategies. My record keeping prompted me to start focusing on marketing campaigns geared toward the difficult-to-reach market, which was later coined, the deconditioned market (a.k.a. couch potatoes). Everyone in those days was focused on the health-and-fitness-conscious consumer and fell impotent when it came to capturing nonusers. I have always believed in the numbers when it comes to business, and the numbers just weren't adding up, because the health-and-fitness-conscious market was so small relative to the overall population. Everyone else was targeting the 8 percent (data in the 1980s) health-and-fitness-conscious and neglecting the 92 percent who were not. I was experiencing so much success with my marketing concepts locally as well as nationally that I couldn't help but think of the obvious progression: I needed to learn how to build a profile of the ideal customer I wanted to focus my marketing efforts toward—the deconditioned consumer with disposable income.

Every now and then, a passing thought would zip through my mind; a voice inside my head would say, "Chuck, you can run promotions on an even larger scale and work with even more clubs." I loved the idea of bringing a ton of new members (and cash) at one time into a health club, but the trick was it had to be done in a way where there would be a future revenue stream from the additional traffic as well. At that point in my life, I was sold on the importance of health and fitness, believing everyone should have the opportunity to be a member of a health club. I knew if I could design a health-club membership with a lower barrier-to-entry by limiting the membership by either days, amenities, or both, I could make the promotion a huge success for everyone. There might not be as much up-front cash, but the back-end revenue would justify the price-point. But then it really hit me: if I could profile the un-committed segment, get them engaged, and then lock up those relationships, I could dwarf the success of any promotion, past or future.

Some portions of my new marketing plan were clear to me within my first few years of selling memberships, but most of the design had been evolving organically through the years. While working as a consultant, I had already persuaded plenty of business owners to start looking to their profit centers (juice bars, tanning beds, personal-training options, and so on) to increase revenue without having to increase membership rates. In fact, most owners were pricing their memberships way too high, diminishing traffic, and therefore the opportunity for their profit centers to thrive. By lowering the barrier-to-entry, we could sell a lot more member-ships and thus have more bodies in the club, which would inevi-tably maximize the profit centers' revenues if promoted correctly through marketing and product placement. At the same time, by making a health-club membership more affordable, I would be opening the doors to a much, much larger audience and could focus my efforts on targeting the nonusers. The fact of the mat-ter was, this concept would only be successful if it penetrated the deconditioned market.

Through trial and error, I developed a more functional sys-tem based on the concept of offering three different classes of memberships at three different price-points using an introduc-tory membership as the draw. The analogy I use when speaking with new club owners is, we're doing exactly what the airline industry has taught us. First-class members pay for first-class ser-vice, business-class members pay for business-class service, and coach-class members pay for and receive coach-class service. They are all going to the same place, just with different levels of service in direct proportion to what they have paid. People want choices. Many retail studies have been done on this subject. Researchers find businesses do best when they offer no more than two or three choices, because anything more is overwhelming to consumers and paralyzes their decision-making processes. Our brains make thousands of choices every day; it is important to keep decision-making to a minimum. This is a fact; do not forget it.

I began jotting down notes and building a business plan. To me, the key was figuring out a way to identify and engage the deconditioned market and study their buying patterns and spending habits as well as their buying triggers. Being out of shape was not the only qualifier; having an interest in health or fitness was just as important. The only way to know their interests was to analyze the consumer's purchases to see if and when, or if they have ever purchased within the health or fitness categories. I wanted to focus our marketing on speaking directly to this audience, which was at least 40 percent of the population at the time.

We already had the attention of the 8–10 percent, the health-and-fitness-conscious, who were receiving attention from all of our competitors. One of the things that amazed me was seeing almost exactly the same marketing pieces from every health club in town. When one club ran a two-for-one offer, everyone ran a two-for-one offer. They all had sexy men and women on their ads, projecting the same images and delivering the same message: this club is for beautiful people who are already fit. Remember what I said about doing what everyone else is doing and what it will get you. It is naïve to believe you can run the exact same offer or campaign your competitor ran and expect the same or better results. The public will respond to whoever was first, but once they see it becoming the norm, they will ignore it just as they do the other sixty-thousand-plus advertisements they see daily. If you want success, you must be the innovator or at least the first to launch the new product or service within your market.

I had been reading about how other industries were looking into market and demographic profiling, confirming my theory there was a way to identify and market to new segments of consumers for any industry. To fully iron out my marketing campaigns, I was also learning about marketing hooks to grab consumers' attention. I knew the cheap price for a basic membership was a great hook from my promotion days, but that was all it could be used for—a hook. I had seen how a fast-food chain offered a free order of fries with any large cheeseburger purchase, and they had people lined up out the door. But people have to know the perceived value of the product first before deciding to stand in line for it. You have to grab consumers' attention and stand out from the thousands of other advertisements in front of them every day. Slowly but surely, I was designing the perfect membership-marketing campaign. It was a good thing, too, because another bomb was about to drop.

I walked in the club one day, and my "partners" told me they had been approached by a couple of top management guys from a national chain that wanted to purchase the clubs (now that I had turned them around and they became competitive in the market). The owners were seriously considering the offer and wanted my opinion. I always try to see what is good about any and every situation in life, so I said, "It's a great idea; especially if you want to get out of the business while you're on top." Inside, I was thinking, this might actually work out best for all parties involved, since I wasn't sure how much longer I would be staying with the four clubs anyway. I immediately asked myself, what's good about this? My brain told me, now you are free to start your own marketing company without feeling guilty about leaving these owners.

In 1989, I reopened CTC (Chuck Thompson Consulting). I did not want to call my company a promotion company, because that reminded me of the fire-sale promotions offered by the promoters

I had worked for in the past, and my vision was to create marketing concepts to ensure the longevity and financial health of all the clubs I represent. I felt I had been building up to this moment since I designed the muscle-head golfer on the cover of my sales-training manual, *Job Security*. My efforts would revolutionize the health-club industry and be a win-win for all. I was determined to build a marketing company that would provide enormous value and I would be paid solely on my performance. I had worked almost my entire life on a success basis (compensated based on my performance), and I wasn't about to stop now. I believe people should be compensated solely on the value they bring to a business. The more value they bring, the higher the compensation should be.

I loved working in those clubs in Chicago. I met a ton of cool people. There have been only two girls in my health-club career, who have gotten away, who I really wanted to date. The first was this little receptionist who worked in the same health club I had started my career in Nashville. She was absolutely beautiful and classy; she dressed like a fashion model and was perfect in my eyes, but at the time, she thought I was too much of a playboy and way too wild for her (which I was). The other was a girl who worked out in one of the clubs in Chicago. Her best friend's boyfriend worked for me as a salesman, and he introduced me to her. I really wanted to date her because she was super sweet and had innocent eyes, a gorgeous smile, and a devilish body. Through our conversations, she discovered I loved playing guitar, and by coincidence, she had previously worked as a backup singer for a legendary blues guitarist. One day, she approached me and said that the bluesman was giving a concert in the city and asked whether I wanted to go. I said hell yeah. She continued to tell me she was going to go backstage before the show and would have him give me an autographed picture. Immediately, I thought, Aw, no!

In the health-club business, I have met more celebrities than most people who are in show business, sports, or even the music business have. I am not star struck, because I know everyone is just a person, just like you and me. It is my firm belief any person can be great if he or she just focuses his or her energy, so I have never been one to take pictures or get autographs; it's just not my thing. I love meeting successful people, not because of their celebrity but because they are at the top of their field. I am just as happy meeting successful businesspeople, inventors, doctors, as I am entertainers. That's why I have avoided dropping celebrities' names in this book. But I am a huge fan of beautiful women, and I knew what I would be doing with her backstage if she were coming to see me, and I just couldn't have that thought in my mind throughout the date, whether anything happened or not; the thought would still be there. I quickly said, "Great, so I'll get to meet so-and-so." She looked at me with those gorgeous eyes and sadly said she was sorry, but I couldn't go with her backstage; I would need to wait for her outside. She thought I was disappointed I wouldn't be meeting the guitar player, but that was the furthest thing from my mind. I couldn't have cared less about him; I just couldn't sit outside while they would be having only God knows what kind of reunion inside his dressing room. The next day, my salesman told me I screwed up big time, because she was dressed to kill that night, and they had partied their asses off. Oh well, things always work out for the best. And the same can be said about my moving away from those clubs and on to the next chapter in my life.

Before I move on, let me share a dozen of the low-cost ways I used to grow the clubs I represented during that time in my career. These tools will be great for you too to generate revenue for your club or your health-and-fitness product. I decided it would be best to finish this chapter by reviewing the lowest-cost marketing tools possible—prospecting and lead generation—because once again in my career I was moving on to a different chapter taking me out of the day-to-day operations and would no longer use most of these rudimentary tools.

I am going to discuss the old as well as the new tools for bringing in business, because when your livelihood and the financial health of a business depend on your ability to generate revenue, you'd better have some inexpensive ways to do it. We will also look at the least expensive ways to market your health club, starting with the Internet and ending with mail-outs. I will give you the pros and cons of each media and platform while teaching you some practical (real-world) applications for all of them. This way, you can hit the ground running no matter what the limitations of your budget may be.

The remainder of this chapter contains what are probably the most important tools and resources for those of you just starting your career, business, or are operating a business, because you can always assume there is no—or at best, a very limited—marketing budget. By coming into a situation with your eyes wide open and with no expectations of help, you'll be prepared for any scenario. Growing the business is the bottom line. The tools I have laid out in this chapter are inexpensive and reliable. Just do your best every day to plant the seeds for generating leads, and I promise you, just as with compound interest, your compensation for your efforts will multiply beyond your wildest expectations. When I first started my consulting career, I had no idea how to run, much less pay for, a full-scale campaign; I busted my butt every day to bring in every dollar from hard work and determination. I am very fortunate, though, because I always find a way to have fun even during difficult times doing the most mundane tasks. The first rule of thumb is ABP: always be prospecting. It's a play on the ABCs of sales: always be closing. Until you have warm bodies in front of you, it's impossible to be closing. Start by having specific prospecting goals and work your way backward through your numbers.

For example, I need to make five sales this week. If my closing ratio is 10 percent of the people I see, then I need to get in front of fifty people this week. If I work five days per week, I need ten solid appointments per day—it's simple math. I can assure you if you consistently have ten confirmed appointments every day, your sales will be far greater than five per week because your closing percentage will skyrocket with all of the practice. It's like anything else in life: the more practice you put in, the better you will inevitably become.

Here are twelve low-cost ways to generate revenue:

1. Buddy sheet: Hands down the easiest, cheapest, and fastest tool is your buddy sheet (or referral sheet). The buddy sheet is designed to help you get contacts with minimal effort. The majority of the work is already done while the process of giving referrals is simplified for the member. The buddy sheet has a list of potential referrals: best friend, brother, sister, aunt, uncle, church friend, and so on. The form is designed this way because when people are approached by someone for a referral, they tend to have a mental hiccup and can't (or don't want to) think of anyone. The buddy sheet takes the thinking out of the equation because it reminds prospects of their friends, neighbors, relatives, and so on.

Most membership directors think of getting referrals only after a sale. I think of getting referrals anytime I speak with anyone. As I said earlier in this book, I built my initial reputation in this business on consistently doubling or tripling a club's gross with no marketing or advertising budget whatsoever. Owners seldom hire a consultant when things are going well; sadly, they are more likely to wait until the business is knocking on death's door. So, asking for a marketing budget was out of the question. As I honed my skills, I designed all of my campaigns around self-funding principles to prove my value to an owner.

The reason I tell you this is because I want you to understand getting referrals was the very first thing I did when I went into a new health club and it didn't cost me a dime. I would always pick up five or ten memberships in just the first day or two and blow everyone's mind. It was as though two audiences were watching two different movies in the same theater. The other salespeople were captivated by what I was accomplishing, and I was horrified by their not doing the same thing a long time ago.

I would simply photocopy a stack of the buddy sheets and stand at the front desk where members checked in. I would smile, introduce myself, welcome them to the club, hand them the sheet, and say, "Please fill this out, and I will give your friends a free one-week pass to train with you."

I did not ask people, "Will you fill it out?" This would have given them the opportunity to say no. I also didn't want them to feel as though they were doing me a favor; I wanted the member to know I was doing them a favor by giving their friends a free one-week pass.

At the end of my first day, I would have hundreds of people to call the following day. Today, it is so much easier with text messaging. Text messaging (SMS) is one of the best platforms for staying in touch with prospects in today's world because everyone carries a mobile device. There are stats that say almost 80 percent of all text messages are read. MMC®'s studies show the real number to be closer to 60 percent, but that is still huge. The downside of text messaging is building a prospect list, since it is an opt-in form of marketing, but for confirming appointments and following up on previous conversations, there is no better platform. The great thing about the buddy sheet is you are getting numbers from family members and friends, so start building your SMS list today.

Another thing about the buddy sheet is that normally a couple of the contacts are very good leads. It is so true that birds of a feather flock together; most people tend to socialize with people in the same income bracket. People who love football tend to socialize with others who love football.

Buddy sheets can also be useful in numerous other ways. You can go to all the businesses around your club and hand them out and tell everyone who fills it out with five good names along with his or her contact information will receive a free thirty-day pass; of course, you better get this strategy approved by your higher-ups beforehand. Again, not all of these leads might pan out, but every time a guest comes in with your pass, you have another opportunity to make more money. This also gives you the chance to sell the guest a membership by giving him or her a special offer or discount, like a first-visit incentive, for trading in the pass and joining today; you may waive the enrollment fee if he or she chooses to join today.

Of course, the most obvious way to use a buddy sheet is after a sale, while the new member is still on an emotional high from taking the first step toward changing his or her life. Just understand that the only limit to a buddy sheet is the limitation of your imagination. Coworkers will look at you funny in the beginning when they first see you using these techniques to get referrals, but later, they will ask you for advice. Never follow the herd; they will take you straight to the slaughterhouse. Always be thinking outside the box, and go for it!

Even if you are unable to close a sale (lock up the relationship), after the presentation, ask for referrals. In most cases, people will gladly give you a name or two, thinking they are refocusing your attention on someone else. Either way, it's a win-win.

2. Guest passes: Wow, again, what a wonderful time to be in the health-and-fitness industry. Back in the day, you had to jump in your car and drive across town to a commercial printer, look through a catalog, pick the font and style of the business card you liked, go back in three days to approve the layout, then go back yet again for corrections if needed, and then finally, go back in a week or two to pick up the cards. Today, you can print high-quality business cards in the comfort of your own home, and if you don't

have a printer at home, you can go to a quick-print shop and have them printed and in your hands within an hour.

In the health-club business, your business cards and guest passes should be one and the same. Print as many as you can afford, and print "one free week" on the back in bright-red letters, along with an expiration date. Carry a bunch of cards in your pocket at all times. Give one to everyone you meet; everyone loves to get something free. This is a great way to socialize as well. When you meet people, introduce yourself and let them know you work at a health club nearby and would be happy to give them a free training session; everyone loves the word "free," especially if the free product or service has real monetary value.

It is very important to include an expiration date to create a sense of urgency. Most people have a tendency to put off until tomorrow what they could have (or should have) done today. We live in a world of procrastinators. Unfortunately for them, but fortunately for us (professional salespeople), they need someone to help them realize their own inner motivations to get started today. There have been numerous studies done on scarcity and how it gets people to take action. For example, if there is only one item left, everyone wants it. But if the item is plentiful, people will say to themselves, "I'll get one later."

When you go to a market, car wash, gas station, restaurant, and so on, you should be handing out guest passes. Every time you give one out, always put the person's name on the pass, and then put their name and mobile number in your lead folder on your smartphone. I cannot express how important building a database of potential clients really is.

Another way to use your business cards is after every sales presentation. I say "every" sales presentation because people tend to forget about referrals and future sales from the prospects who do not buy (a.k.a. prospects who walk). Every prospect you visit with, should walk away with two guest passes, and you should walk away with two fresh leads. Some people will not want the paper in this paperless world, but you should always have cards readily available because it will at least give you something tangible to give prospects. Also, have a guest pass on your smartphone so you can Bluetooth them to prospects as well.

So far, I have talked about two fantastic ways to get started on generating sales with just a couple of bucks invested in paper and ink. Now that you have sold a couple of memberships, it's time you start investing in your future. Again, I will start out with low-budget ways of generating leads before discussing more costly mediums.

3. Lead boxes: Lead boxes are also called registration boxes. I know some of you out there are going to think these three resources (i.e., buddy sheets, guest passes, and lead boxes) are old school, and they are, but they work. If you want to be great, you have to be willing to do the things others won't, old school or new. I must also warn you that the laws have changed drastically since I was in the field using lead boxes, and you must check with your club's owner (and he or she with an attorney) on the current laws regarding this matter. I know there will definitely be a ratio of winners based on number of registrants. Back in the day, some owners used to put pictures of tropical settings on their boxes, which read, "Win a free trip to the Bahamas." That was totally misleading because those trips were set up by real-estate companies selling timeshare condo units. The winners had to sit through a weekend-long sales presentation instead of spending all day in the sand as they had hoped. When I put out lead boxes on my own, I just used a picture of a sexy girl and guy on the top and wrote "win a free one-year health-club membership" above the picture, and I always got a great response.

If you're working for a club, ask the owner to buy a hundred boxes for the business; they're very cheap, and they pay high dividends. If the owner buys them, of course he or she will put the club's logo and name on them, and they will be his or her property. If he or she will not buy them, get permission in writing to do it yourself, and ask whether you can get a higher commission on your sales to offset your investment. The worst thing the owner can say is no, but you'll never know until you ask. If you buy the boxes, they're your property, and you can design them however you wish. Don't include the club's name or logo unless it's easy to change; this way if you leave or start your own club, you will have a head start on your marketing materials. Also put on the box that all registrants will win a free one-week pass to such-and-such health club just for registering.

The most important things to remember with lead boxes are the three laws of real estate: location, location, and location. Map out your marketplace, and find the top fifty locations with the highest volume of traffic (preferably related to health and fitness); then make a list of the second highest, third highest, and so on. Then call each store to get the GM's name and schedule.

Next load your car up with the boxes on your days off, and drive to the businesses (or walk if you have to—I did when I first started). Most people will tell you to call to set an appointment first, and I agree it would be more polite, but the reality is most people will tell you no over the phone as a knee-jerk response before they ever hear your proposition. I repeat: put the boxes out on your days off. You don't want to leave the club on workdays because you could miss a sale.

Walk into the store carrying the box in your arms where everyone can see it (preferably wearing your uniform if you have one), and ask to speak to the GM. I used to wear my uniform almost every day, not just because I was poor, although that may have been a contributing factor. We had these cool dark-blue-silk Adidas warmup suits (remember that it was the early 1980s), and I bought one for every day. I got the idea because when I went to lunch, someone would inevitably ask me about the health club because of the logo on my name tag, and I generated a ton of leads that way. My coworkers thought I was crazy for keeping my name tag on, but I didn't care about what they thought; they weren't paying my bills. They would barely wear their name tags inside the club because they thought they were too cool for name tags. I thought they were being silly because it cost them business.

After being introduced to the manager of the store where you want to place your lead box, let him or her know the purpose of the visit. Explain you would like to put a registration box near the entrance or exit so all of the store's customers can receive a free one-week pass to your health club, and just for letting you do this, you'll give him or her a free membership for as long as the box stays in the store and is producing. Make sure the managers understand (and you do too) they are VIPs as far as you are concerned and you plan on taking very good care of them when they are in your club. You must take good care of the GMs who say yes because their experiences in your club will motivate them to generate tons of business for you by encouraging their patrons to register.

Now is a great time to introduce the fact that there are five basic things on most people's minds when conducting business or listening to business presentations:

1. What is the product or service?
2. What's in it for me, that is, what problem will it solve?
3. What's your proof?
4. Why do I need the product or service now?
5. Which emotional need will the product or service fulfill?

I have said the following many times, and I will repeat it throughout this book: people buy for emotional reasons and justify their purchases with logical reasons. So, give the GM emotional reasons to partner with you, like connection, importance, contribution, and by giving all of his or her customers a free one-week pass he or she can logically justify displaying the box. Don't expect everyone to say yes, because not everyone will. Sales is a numbers game; that's why I told you to start with your *A* prospects (top fifty), then *B* (second fifty), *C* (third fifty), and so on. If you have twenty boxes to put out in a day, you might have to visit two hundred stores, but if you are persistent and do your homework, you will succeed.

After collecting your leads, call them all and invite them in for free workouts. I always had several guys and gals around the club who loved training people but hated the sales process, so I would make a deal with them where I would set up potential members with training appointments during the trainers' downtimes, and they would train my prospects for one thirty-minute session for free. This was a win-win for everyone. The prospect received a personal-training session (with a value of at least twenty dollars), the trainer had a new prospect, and I sold another membership.

4. Cold calls: Cold calling is also called telemarketing or dialing for dollars. The laws regarding telemarketing have changed dramatically as well as with lead boxes, so be sure to check with your club's owner or an attorney before you start dialing for dollars. In the old days, sales counselors could grab the white pages (yellow pages were for business listings, and white pages were for residential listings) and just start hammering out calls. The phone companies even had little neighborhood directories, so salespeople could stay within their market; of course, all of this research to find local residents' telephone numbers can be done online now. I use the word "we" loosely because most membership counselors hated to get on the phone to make cold calls. I never understood their reluctance. I would hear them complaining about their car payments, their rents being past due, and their lack of sales, yet they would just cry on the shoulder of whoever would listen instead of picking up the phone.

All sales-training methods will tell you to qualify the prospect: First, does he or she have the money to buy a membership? I agree with qualifying your prospects 99 percent of the time, especially if you are spending marketing dollars, but there are always exceptions to every rule. So, don't give up on your prospect if he or she is jobless. You might be able to get that person to work for you by bringing you a new prospect every time he or she comes to the club to train.

One time I was in the club in Nashville, and a prospect came in wearing overalls and work boots. This was in the very beginning of my career, and I don't think I was even on the up list (a list made by the sales manager to determine who would get the first shot at walk-in—prospects that come in unexpectedly without being solicited by one of the sales staff). When the other guys saw this older farmer, they made a beeline to the offices; no one wanted to tour him around but me. I asked whether they would mind if I gave it a shot, and laughingly, they all gave me their blessings. They all thought that old-timer would never join, because he looked as though he just stepped down off a tractor; later, I found out that he literally had just gotten off his tractor.

I learned he had just left a tobacco auction after selling his tobacco crop and came in to see us because his doctor told him to start exercising or he would die; that was powerful leverage to move him to take action immediately. One of the greatest tools available to move something or someone is leverage. Earlier, when discussing sales presentations, I discussed how to create leverage and how to use that leverage to move a prospect to take immediate action. Doctors have a great handle on this concept by using the fear of death as a lever. It worked on this tobacco farmer, and he came in with a pocketful of cash.

Health clubs used to sell lifetime memberships with a ridiculously low guaranteed-renewal fee per year after the initial term of the membership expired. This was a great sales tool since a lot of people liked paying once and never worrying about it again. The health-club owners loved it too because it brought in a nice chunk of change every year from renewals, until lifetime memberships were outlawed.

After spending some time with the farmer and getting him engaged and emotionally connected with the club, along with the doctor's leverage, which motivated him to buy, I sold him a lifetime membership, and he paid cash in full. This was a huge deal for me because our commission for a PIF membership (paid in full) was much larger than for a financed membership. I think I made a couple hundred dollars on that one sale since the membership cost around $2,000. Man, the other membership directors were pissed at themselves. They had judged the book by its coveralls. So, never assume anything, and go through each sales presentation from *A* to *Z* no matter whom you are presenting. In my opinion, everyone is a qualified prospect if you take the time to learn how he or she qualifies, and if you are just starting out in business, you have the time to present your product to everyone who is willing to listen. Later, I will go into detail about prequalifying prospects before wasting your advertising dollars, but for a membership director who is new to the business, you just need warm bodies in front of you.

Never try to sell anything over the phone (unless that's the primary way your product or service is sold), but the appointment is the rule to remember when cold calling; this is where I think novices get discouraged. People get caught up in long conversations on the phone and end up justifying their products or services instead of getting the consumer excited about an appointment. It is difficult (not impossible) to get prospects' emotions and senses engaged over the phone, but if they're face-to-face in your club, it is easy. So, get them off the phone and into the club.

There are cold calls made by machines, called robocalls. During any election year, you will receive these at your home, but only politicians and emergency agencies are allowed to use them. There have been numerous laws passed lately with huge fines if you're robocalling people on their home phones, and now, some states have even made it illegal to robocall mobile phones. Stay far away from this type of telemarketing, because you will regret it.

5. Corporate cold calls: Dialing for dollars can also be used to grow relationships with local businesses. Call them, and invite them in for a free training session for all of their employees or executives. It can be set up as a field trip or company function or a health-and-fitness awareness day. It can be presented to the employees as a gift from their company, earning goodwill for the employer. I hope I do not need to say it again at this point, but you will be building your list of prospects with every contact you make.

Before you start making your calls, do your homework:

- Know who the prospect is, and get as much information as possible about the prospect, which is a little more difficult when you're dialing for dollars just to get appointments, but when you're calling businesses, you need to get to the decision-makers and get their attention immediately.

  When speaking with your prospects, identify ASAP whether they are the decision-makers or gatekeepers. If they are the gatekeeper (usually these are secretaries who block unwanted calls, including sales calls) or not the decision-makers, direct your presentation to their needs as well as their bosses, since this is a bridge you must successfully cross before getting to the decision-maker.

  Anticipate some of his or her wants, needs, or pain points. What are his or her interests? Most secretaries know more about their bosses' schedules than their bosses do. Secretaries are the perfect candidates for flowers, candies, Christmas cards, birthday cards, and e-mails; add them to your Facebook, Snapchat, Twitter, and other social-media accounts. You must get on the good side of the secretaries because they will be the ones to get you in front of their bosses.

- Learn as much as possible about the person you will be meeting with before you go to the appointment. This is especially important for corporate cold calls. Find something you have in common, like a sport, cars, food, or arts. Discover what you like about the person you're meeting with so you can pay him or her a sincere compliment. Make a list of questions you can ask before arriving at the business for the appointment, both pain and pleasure questions.

The more questions your prospect asks about your health club, the more interested he or she is. The same goes for you too; the more relevant questions you ask your prospects, the more interested you will seem. Take a few minutes, write down a bunch of questions to ask your prospects that are relevant to their likes and dislikes, and put them in your quiver to use in future conversations; I promise they will serve you well.

Think of, and address prospects' wants and needs. If you address their needs, they will take the conversation to the next level. When probing, always remember prospects' first answers may be knee-jerk reaction, such as, "I don't have the time to go to a health club," but a couple of follow-up questions may reveal the true reasons for the pushback.

When you are preparing to make your calls, prepare yourself for rejection. It is an inevitable fact of life, especially in sales. The greatest ballplayers of all time get hits about every three times at bat, and the greatest salespeople close about the same percentage of cold-call prospects as well (you are not a professional cold caller, so don't beat yourself up if you can't close 30 percent of your calls). The easiest way to avoid rejection is to never go for the hard close. What I mean by this is constantly build value and ask test-closing questions along the way. For example, start with, "Which day of the week is best for you and your executives?" as opposed to "Do you want to buy a corporate membership?" If you go for the hard close, you will get a hard yes or no answer, and if it is no, you will be fighting an uphill battle; but if you're just test-closing, you will know whether your prospect is hot or cold.

Another reality you will run into is some of your prospects will already be members of another health club. This is a golden opportunity for you to learn all about the competition. What does the prospect like most and dislike most about his or her health club? Align with what he or she likes, and show how your health club is completely different in reference to the bad; but never bad-mouth the competition. No one is interested in being told he or she made a stupid decision by joining another health club. Just highlight the things you do that no one else does or the things your health club does better than any other club, such as, providing unparalleled customer service.

- Be prepared for objections. Have a minimum of six rebuttals for every possible objection. Know all the possible objections, write down your rebuttals, and commit them to memory. Make it a game, and be excited to overcome them.
- Expect the best; prepare for the worst. Be able to adjust. People will cancel appointments. People won't always do things your way. If someone cancels an appointment, be flexible. Prepare for inevitable setbacks.
- Create demand. It is absolutely imperative there be a demand for your health-and-fitness product or service and that the prospect is aware of that demand.

You need at least ten benefits a prospect will get by giving you an appointment, just as you need ten benefits a prospect will get by joining your health-club today, and ten reasons why your product is worth ten times more than your membership rates.

Outline your phone presentation, and set your goals. I scheduled cold calls for times when I couldn't be doing something that paid bigger and faster dividends. It will be necessary to track your responses from all of your efforts in order to gauge the immediate return on investment (your time). I say this because cold calls are on the lower rung of the ladder for me. I prefer face-to-face meetings anytime, but I also know sometimes, I must step out of my comfort zone to grow and get better, so I try everything.

Set specific goals for your phone calls, and stick to your game plan for your calls, for example, gather information, build rapport, and set an appointment.

When calling a prospect to set an appointment, follow these three easy steps:

1. Let the prospect know what's in it for him or her.
2. State the emotional and logical reasons he or she should meet with you.
3. Give examples of the pain he or she may be experiencing and the pleasure associated with your health-and-fitness product or service, and explain how it will either alleviate or eliminate his or her pain.

When setting an appointment, ask for only ten minutes of his or her time, and guarantee if he or she is not fully interested in what you have to say, you will not take up any more of their time. Everyone can find ten minutes in a day, but no one has twenty minutes. Start with, and be happy with, ten minutes; don't worry, because if he or she likes what you have to say, time will never be an issue.

How many appointments do you want, and how many calls will it take for you to get that number of appointments? What is your hook to get your foot in the door? For example, "I want to give your executives a free day at the club." What area will you call, and what time would be best for calling? What message will you leave if you get a voice mail? You should have a plan to achieve all goals. The next step is to implement your plan, and then adjust to unforeseen challenges. Once you have planned and are prepared, go for it!

6. Comarketing strategies: Partner with your local Chamber of Commerce or other organizations to offer special discounts for their members: police departments, fire departments, municipalities, teachers' unions, and so on. Develop a great corporate offer (using volume pricing), contact all the people you can, and ask them to send out e-mails, put inserts into their newsletters, put the offer on their Facebook page, or any other platform used to stay in contact with members, associates, or affiliates. Make sure your offer is a real value and is a win-win across the board.

7. Social-media platforms: Using social media is paramount for any business, especially businesses that have a social component to them. Facebook's pros: Facebook (FB) has the possibility to get enormous traffic if it is marketed properly. Your FB friends list is another marketing list. FB advertising is cheap and easy. Facebook allows you to post ads even without a website.

Facebook's cons: Facebook has low conversion rates for e-commerce because people use Facebook to communicate with their friends and loved ones and are not expecting to read your ads. Ad clutter is a problem because Facebook allows almost everyone to post ads; your ads may be posted with other irrelevant ads. It is hard to capture your audience's full attention since they are chatting, playing, or doing other activities on Facebook.

One of the other big selling points of Facebook's paid ads is they allow you to profile your targets. This is extremely misleading. Facebook's profiling is rudimentary at best, providing you only four parameters to profile your prospects:

1. Geography (Fantastic, but a lot of people who sign up for Facebook accounts give false information to avoid scammers.)
2. Gender (Fantastic, but a lot of people who sign up for Facebook accounts give false information to avoid scammers.)
3. Age (Fantastic, but a lot of people who sign up for Facebook accounts give false information to avoid scammers.)
4. Interests (Fantastic, but a lot of people who sign up for Facebook accounts give false information to avoid scammers.)

You might think you are advertising to a beautiful brunette with a big smile when you are really targeting a blue-haired seventy-year-old with no teeth (Facebook profiles are notoriously filled with false information). "You get what you pay for" is a saying that resonates for a reason: minimal investments bring less than minimal returns.

Twitter's pros: Twitter allows you to communicate to a large group of people with one message. It is great as a quick communication platform to promote the content of your health club. It is the simplest to use of all the social-media platforms. It's absolutely free.

Twitter's cons: There is a limit to the number of characters allowed, which limits your message. Not all people use or understand Twitter. Twitter can be distracting.

I chose to highlight just Facebook and Twitter as examples, but there are hundreds of social-media platforms. Most of them don't provide enough benefits to justify the time or the effort needed to sign up with them. As far as producing any measurable results when it comes to growing your health club, well, let's just say you have to be patient; it's going to take a while.

You get what you pay for in life, you get back what you put out, and so on. If you are looking to find free health-club marketing platforms, there are some out there. But if you are looking to launch a health-club marketing campaign to grow your health club, you might want to look at media and platforms that are going to produce the desired result.

Social media is great for what it is, but it has yet to evolve into a great tool for marketing health clubs that rely on foot traffic for growing their businesses.

8. E-mail marketing campaigns: E-mail marketing is probably the most misunderstood and enormously abused health-club marketing platform of all. E-mail marketing is often presented as the best way to market health clubs because it is the most effective and least expensive marketing tool available. This couldn't be the further from the truth.

Just as with any other form of marketing, the most important factor is your prospect list. Some health clubs are just now (twenty-five years later than they should have been) building their e-mail lists. Most health clubs have a handful of e-mail addresses primarily from current members. So, most health-club marketing done via e-mail is actually marketing to the existing membership base made up of core members; hence, e-mail marketing does not capture new business in most cases.

E-mail marketing pros: E-mail marketing is affordable or free; the response from the targeted audience is often fast. The customer-tracking ability is great; e-mail marketing campaigns can be launched with ease; and no other delivery system is faster than e-mails. You have the ability to send different e-mails whenever you wish, reaching targeted audiences by customizing e-mail offers based on their interests.

E-mail marketing cons: E-mail marketing is plagued with security and privacy issues. Most clients nowadays have ad-blocking software, most e-mail ads require customers to download a JPEG or PDF file, and some of these ads are large and therefore time-consuming to download. E-mails are sometimes considered unimportant and are often deleted by the audience. Some e-mail ads are hard to read, especially on mobile devices.

Health-club e-marketing is extremely low-cost once you have built a database of qualified recipients because the delivery of your message is free. But if you are not building your list, you are not growing your list, and therefore you are not growing your business. Building a qualified prospect e-mail list is time-consuming and will require a financial investment. Never buy an e-mail list, because it will cause you unmentionable problems with your IP (Internet-protocol) address, your ISP (Internet service provider), your ranking on search engines like Google, Bing, Yahoo and so on; sending out e-mails to a bad list could even get your website blocked or blacklisted.

E-mail marketing is an opt-in form of health-club marketing, so you must build your list in-house. There are no shortcuts to this process, no matter what anyone tries to tell (or sell) you. Even some of the people who have been in the health-club cybermarketing business for years will neglect to tell you the downsides to e-marketing, just to get you to buy their e-mail marketing packages. Not everyone will get caught but for the few that do, it can be devastating.

The CAN-SPAM Act is a law that sets the rules for commercial e-mail, establishes requirements for commercial messages, gives recipients the right to have you stop e-mailing them, and spells out tough penalties for violations.

Here are the penalties for violating the CAN-SPAM Act: Each separate e-mail in violation of the law is subject to penalties of up to $16,000, and more than one person may be held responsible for violations. For example, both the company whose product is promoted in the message and the company that originated the message may be legally responsible. E-mails that make misleading claims about products or services may also be subject to laws outlawing deceptive advertising, like Section 5 of the FTC Act. The

CAN-SPAM Act has certain aggravated violations that may give rise to additional fines. The law provides for criminal penalties, including imprisonment.

Buy e-mails from a third party and send them out or have a third party send them out promoting your products or services to purchased e-mail addresses that have not opted-in at your own risk, but you have been warned. Besides the legalities, it's considered to be unethical in the cyber world.

9. SMS messages: SMS is a fantastic platform for marketing health-and-fitness products and services, but this platform is also far from inexpensive. SMS messaging is inexpensive to deliver if it is being sent from an in-house account, but can be very expensive if controlled by a third party. It also can be extremely expensive to build your SMS list. SMS marketing in relative terms can be either extremely expensive or inexpensive, depending on whether you are starting with a qualified list of mobile numbers.

If you do not have a quality list to start with, you must first launch an initial marketing campaign via radio, print, direct mail, and so on just to build the list of mobile-phone numbers you'll need for an SMS marketing campaign. SMS marketing is an opt-in form of marketing, so you must get the prospects' permission first before messaging them.

SMS marketing also demands you keep your messages short and sweet. This requires a lot of knowledge of the psychology of health-club marketing.

With that said, SMS is absolutely a great support platform for your marketing campaigns, and if you are smart, you will begin to capture mobile numbers immediately, so when the time comes for you to launch an SMS marketing campaign, you will be prepared. Everything is being condensed to fit on mobile devices, so be prepared to keep your message to the point when it comes to mobile marketing. One day in the near future, it will be an excellent way to engage prospects, but for now, it is dependent on other media to first capture your prospects' pertinent information and permission.

10. Content-marketing options: You must design a professional website where you give free information to the public about health and fitness every week. Send out free newsletters (not sales brochures) and articles that give instruction and education on health and fitness. You can also send out free survey results, free data, and so on. Informational and educational content is today's way of selling. The information highway is exactly that—a highway for information to travel on. Consumers have become accustomed to using the Internet to research health products and health-club services. Providing premium content is an excellent way to start conversations and relationships with prospects and members.

Another tool for content marketing would be to put something of great value, like a free download, on your website as a reward to anyone who registers with your website, and then take those who register to a second step of the sales process, which could be having them read your blog posts and so on. Take people through a sales presentation without emphasizing sales. It is your job to engage consumers and keep them engaged with valuable content. Freebies and bonuses are also excellent ways of doing this. Show your visitors you are just as interested in serving as you are in selling.

11. Flyers: Most of us just starting out can't afford to pay for direct mail, but we can photocopy flyers and put them in mailboxes around our neighborhoods. Make it fun, and incorporate it into your exercise regimen. Walk, and put out flyers for an hour every day. There are companies that specialize in this business of putting out door hangers. They hire people for minimum wage to hang advertising on doorknobs. If you can't afford to pay for advertising, get out, and start walking.

12. Mail-outs: Birthday cards, Christmas cards, motivational postcards, invitational letters, and so on are all great ways to follow

up with prospects you have just spoken with over the phone or met briefly. Everyone wants (and needs) to feel special, whether he or she will admit it or not, and tangible-correspondence meets this need far better than an e-mail or other digital communication; mail-outs are a great way to stay connected. Remember in the sales presentation when I discussed the four different social styles: the director, the analytical, the socialist, and the relator. Your prospect's dominant social style and preferred communication style, will be the dictating factors of your follow-up method. With directors, who are only concerned with the bottom line in the beginning, you do not want to call them all of the time to follow up, because they will inevitably get annoyed by your interruptions and blow you off for good. Handwritten (legible) cards are perfect for this scenario and occasional follow-up calls. On the other hand, if your prospect is a socialist, a phone call would be expected. Socialists love the connection and look forward to and welcome new relationships. A relator will need a list of testimonials, and an analytical will want all the details in writing. People like people like themselves; do not forget this fact, follow the prospect's style of preferred communication and not yours.

If you are just fishing for prospects and have not spent enough time with someone to determine his or her preferred style of communication or social style, then use the shotgun method until you find what works best. Always keep a budget for mail-outs. You have an exact bull's-eye on qualified prospects; it's personal, tangible, and direct.

Again, set your goals with your desired outcome, do your homework, design your presentation pieces, ad copy, decide on your hook and go for it!

I have just given you a dozen low-cost ways to bring in new business. You don't have to use them all (although you should), but even if you use just a few, you will have a few more opportunities every day to make a sale. One of my favorite sayings is "Luck is when preparation meets opportunity." Always be prepared.

Health-club marketing and professional health-club membership sales go hand in hand. One of the things most talked about within the sales community is leads. Whether they are cold or hot, qualified or not, the bottom line is, if you have a warm body with the money to join your club, you have a smokin' hot sales lead. I have never looked at prospects in front of me, or referral from my members, or guys who are brought in by a member to work out as my only hot leads. Don't take what I am saying the wrong way; those referrals and walk-ins are great leads and definitely qualify as hot leads. But buddy referrals and walk-ins are not your only sources of hot leads. Just think about it: everybody in your community is theoretically a hot lead, so go out and get 'em to come in and take a tour of your magnificent club today.

CHAPTER 6

PUTTING ALL THE PIECES TOGETHER

I t was 1989, and I was twenty-six years young, I had been in the health-club business approximately seven years. I started in sales and worked my way through lower management, to middle management, to upper management, and to so-called partial ownership. I had been a consultant for numerous clubs on operations, sales, marketing, and I had written a manual on professional membership sales. By this time in my career, I had probably sold or been directly responsible for selling well over 250,000 club memberships. I was now going to invest everything I had and market health clubs my way. My goal was to identify, engage, and then lock up relationships with the difficult-to-reach market known as the deconditioned (couch potatoes) market. If I succeeded or fell flat on my face, it would all be on me, and I was ready for the challenge.

Subconsciously, I had been preparing for that day my entire life. I had studied every facet of the health-club industry. I was a sponge that absorbed every ounce of pertinent information relative to increasing revenue and sales. For the past several years, I had been raising hundreds of thousands of dollars a month for privately owned and operated clubs, and now, I was going to do it on a mass scale. I could have gone into any single health club, and worked my butt off twelve hours a day, seven days a week for thirty days, and increased the club's revenue drastically, but I would be limited to helping twelve clubs a year, and inevitably, those clubs would go back to their old ways and habits of running a business as soon as I left. Not to mention I would be doing the same thing over and over, like a hamster on a wheel, and if you know anything about me by now, you know I cherish variety and growth. Besides, I wanted to create a product that would carry a club for two to three years, which would be long enough for the owners and management to cultivate relationships with the new members and earn their long-term loyalty.

I first needed to do my research. The first place everyone should start when building a business or career is research. As I said previously, I wanted to target a much larger market than was currently being addressed—the deconditioned market. From experience, it was crystal clear to me no one was tapping into this segment because no one knew how to identify who they were or, even harder, how to get them in the door. Most people who buy health clubs, gyms, spas, fitness centers, athletic clubs, and racquet clubs normally have an emotional tie to health and fitness or a specific sport but very little working knowledge of the business. Normally, its doctors, lawyers, athletes, muscle heads, fitness fanatics, and so on, who love to train or love nutrition, who have an epiphany one day and think, I should open a health club?

It is the entrepreneur's love for the sport, activity or lifestyle that blinds them from the reality—and in some cases the nightmare—of running a health club like a business. That is, of course, until their entire life savings have been depleted and the bank won't float them any more loans. Up until then, they suffer from the *Field of Dreams* delusion: build it, and they shall come. Had they done only the most basic research, they would have known that about 10 percent (now as high as 20 percent in 2016) of the population in the United States are health-and-fitness-conscious, 20 percent are health-and-fitness aware, and today, almost 60 percent are still the polar opposite of health-and-fitness-conscious, with more than 30 percent being borderline obese.

Here is a quick formula you can use to see whether you should open a health club in a particular area or neighborhood. Please keep in mind there's a lot of factors that must be considered, and use this simple matrix as just a starting point. Put your proposed location into Google Maps and draw three-, five-, seven-, and ten-mile circles around it. Do not BS yourself; accurately determine how far people will drive to train at a club in your geographical area. If the club is downtown or in a big city, maybe they'll drive one block to one mile; if it's suburbia with heavy traffic, maybe three to five miles; if it's rural, maybe five to seven miles; and if it's deep in the country, seven to twenty miles at best, but never estimate more than twenty miles. In short, the travel time should be no longer than fifteen to twenty minutes.

Next, look at the number of households (not number of people), and take 15 percent of that number, and you will have a calculated guess as to the number of potential members that a health club can draw from your geographical area. Let me address two things at this point: why households and not population, and why I say 15 percent and not 20 percent. I have been conducting health-club research since the 1980s, and although today's consumers are far more educated about health and fitness, I always prefer to err on the conservative side. So, with my formula, you might be happily surprised but not devastated by overinflated hope and unrealistic numbers. Besides, the kids in a household may be health-and-fitness conscious but not in the market for a health-club membership. Of course, there are bonus prospects who drive by your club on their way to and from work, or who live a little farther out, but do not factor these prospects into your equation.

You and every other health-and-fitness business in that radius will be competing for that 15 percent, so do not be fooled, as so many before you have been, by thinking the little gym down the street is not competition. If it has even one person giving the business as little as one dollar, it is your competition, because that one body came from the 15 percent. Learn everything you can about every aerobics center, Pilates center, fitness center, health club, athletic club, YMCA, and so on within your market, and go visit them all. Ask them questions about their memberships and their membership rates, sit through and actively listen to their sales presentations, go back several times—especially on Monday and Tuesday evenings around six p.m. and look at their parking lot to see how crowded they are. Go in for a workout as a guest, and ask some of the staff how many members they have. You can even try to guess (because that is really all you can do at this stage of your research) how many members each club has based on its Monday and Tuesday evening workouts, and how many cars are in the parking lot between 4:00 p.m. and 8:00 p.m. if you can't get a number from one of the staff.

The health-club business is all about the numbers. Fifty percent of the people who join a club never come back, even to pick up their membership cards; another 30 percent drop-off in the first six months. These numbers are based on averages from all across the United States and will vary from club to club, but they are close enough for you to gauge the feasibility of opening a club in the market you have chosen as a start-up business with limited resources. At least you'll be able to make some educated guesses.

Take your 15 percent of households, which will give you your potential market, and then subtract the possible members enrolled with your competition, remove them from your total, and now you have a realistic number of potential members for your club. Keep in mind I haven't discussed all of the variables that could catapult your membership numbers far beyond the norm: for example, you own a niche portion of the market, your service is unparalleled, you are the most convenient, your amenities blow the competition away, you have a top-notch, well-trained membership-sales staff using a professional-sales system, you're in a freestanding building, you're on the ground level of a shopping center, your marketing company works twenty-four hours a day, seven days a week promoting your health club as well as your health-and-fitness products and services, and so on. I am just talking hard, raw basic numbers.

A second must is to determine whether your market will support your projected price-point. I always get a kick out of owners when we are in a meeting discussing membership marketing concepts, and they tell me their best market is a neighborhood twenty minutes away. They normally say this because it is a higher income area, and they want to pull from that area because they fantasize it is their demographic. They will even sometimes say, "I live there, and I drive here every day." And I reply "Well, you drive here every day because you have your entire life's savings or credit rating tied up in this place; prospects don't share the same motivation as you." You can absolutely pull those people from there, but it takes a lot more than simple desire. In fact, it takes a lot of know-how, patience, and you must create a need and desire for customers to drive the extra distance. But I want to give you tools you can put to use today, right now. So, my advice is to focus on your immediate area and price your memberships based on the demographic makeup of your local market and not on the demographic makeup of your wish list of prospects. Later, you can partner with a professional health-club marketing company like MMC® to assist you in capturing your desired market.

As I was saying, I too wanted to research my targeted audience before I even attempted to approach a health-club owner about running a campaign. I had seen endless owners struggle with their marketing, and in my opinion, it was mostly because of their misdirected ads. They went after the same market their competitors went after—the health-and-fitness-conscious. Everyone was seeing the same ads with the same offers all the time. I knew if I was going to be successful, I would have to build a profile of my clients' ideal customer, and that is exactly what I did.

Back then (in 1989), the Internet had just hit the market, and I was the furthest thing from a computer geek, so I did my research the old-fashioned way—by talking to customers, and paying a fortune to companies to gather the data for me. By the way, talking to your existing members and prospects will give you some of the best free information, education, and data you can ever obtain. The research I am referring to is called primary research. Primary research is custom-designed (by yourself or a company you hire) for the particular needs of a company like MMC® to profile the ideal customer for their clients and is often conducted by professional researchers, but in today's world of the Internet, the research can also be done by individuals if they have the time to devote to learning the craft. This is necessary research if you plan on growing your business or career, especially as a marketer. I will discuss in some detail the process of what I did while explaining some of the end results I was looking for, so you too may apply some of the same techniques to your business's research as well.

First, you need to think of research in two ways:

1. Member's attitudes—emotions and feelings
2. Member's behaviors—buying patterns and spending habits

You start primary research by listening to your members and not to yourself. Suspend your ego temporarily, and get the information you need from the source—your members. Your members have a wealth of information just waiting to be harvested; they will tell you why they are happy, sad, disappointed, and pleased; why they joined; why they didn't join your competitor; and why they stay or, worse, why they are planning to leave.

In my situation, my team and I interviewed hundreds of members and nonmembers alike. I wanted to know why certain people loved being members of their local health clubs yet others never joined. What were their fears, what media caught their attention, what did they read or just toss, what programs did they watch, what made them flip the channel, what were the psychological triggers that made them not buy, and what were the triggers that made them buy? A lot of marketers miss the boat when it comes to demographic research because they only focus on income and age—which are two of the most basic qualifiers that fall at the very bottom of a comprehensive consumer profile. Keep in mind when members (consumers) are asked questions about a product or service, their knee-jerk response is normally price. When digging a little deeper during a personal one-on-one interview or small group setting, you'll find that this isn't always the real challenge that must be addressed and overcome. If you ask some simple questions, you will uncover unmet needs, wants, wishes, and desires, and then you can design a way to identify those consumers as a group. The realities of the marketplace can force you to rethink your position and priorities, so you must know your target audience like the back of your hand before launching a new product.

Today, there is a ton of information readily available via the Internet. There has been a global explosion of consumer-behavior information available to anyone who is willing to invest the time and personnel to find it. Massive databases allow marketers access to credit-card spending patterns, consumers' purchase habits, and demographic data that is even broken down by zip codes, neighborhoods, and street addresses. You (anyone with the time, a clear objective, and Internet access) can also unearth or purchase data about members from numerous sources on the Internet that is not easily surrendered by participants who take part in surveys or focus groups. Some of this information is even free. The process of gathering the data and interpreting the information is time-consuming, but if you have more time than money, it is definitely an option.

Market research has always been at the top of my list and is now MMC®'s top priority. When I was building this company, and even during its inception, my focus was on the members. Throughout this book, I use the term "win-win"; this is the guiding principle of my life. If members can feel like winners by joining my clients' health clubs as opposed to their competitors', they will feel more connected to the club; which in turn, will inspire member loyalty. This philosophy creates the ultimate win-win relationship, so I took my research a lot deeper than first anticipated, before I ever considered launching this new member-acquisition campaign.

My goal was, and still is, to define our client's target audience on a national scale, so we dug deeper and deeper to unearth as much applicable information as possible. We researched consumers' psychographics including attitudes, beliefs, perceptions, lifestyles, personality traits, as well as frequencies of purchase, frequencies of use of a product or service within the health and fitness categories, volumes of purchase, rates of use, occasions of use, brand loyalties, price sensitivities, price levels, buying situations or occasions, demographics, geographic areas, and on and on.

I contracted a lot of people and companies to help with this process, and this research is still ongoing even today. MMC®'s team of researchers is gathering new data daily for all of our clients. Any given project has up to thirty people devoted to its success. In the late 1980s, I had to purchase all of this data from outside sources, and through decades of experience and hundreds of thousands of dollars invested, I eventually learned how to conduct more detailed research specific to MMC®'s needs as health-club marketers, so later in my career when I could afford it, I built a research center where we employ an entire department that works twenty-four hours a day, seven days a week, gathering and interpreting data for our clients. After profiling my ideal target, I needed to design ad copy that focused on getting targets (prospects and guests) through the door. I set out to accomplish this through perfecting my message and offer.

It's important to understand psychology as it relates to selling health-club memberships, health-and-fitness products, and health-and-fitness services. Knowing the needs and wants of your audience and how your health-and-fitness product can satisfy them is critical to your success. You might work out because it makes you feel successful. Some people work out because it allows them to connect with their friends; others because it helps them build new relationships or rekindle old relationships; some because it is challenging, and they are excited to see results in the mirror; and some because it makes them feel good. Never be fooled into believing your customers join for the same reasons. There are, however, a core set of reasons or emotions that can explain 80 percent of your prospects' buying decisions.

You must know what emotion(s) the customer in front of you is chasing, so you can let him or her experience that feeling right then which will start the process of him or her linking extreme pleasure to your product or service. Try to think about the value of your brand in terms of its emotional equity—how your health club, product or service makes your prospects and members feel. The biggest mistake we can make is to think every guest or member comes through our doors for the same reason(s) or is interested in our product or service for the same reason(s) we are.

Part of my focus, and now MMC®'s focus, is on meeting the six core emotional needs of the consumer in our advertising as well as in our sales presentations. Security, importance, excitement, connection, growth, and contribution are all emotional needs that must be connected with your health-and-fitness product or service and conveyed through your marketing and sales systems. Once I knew my target (the deconditioned consumers) market I had to design my advertising to trigger their core emotional needs.

The word "member" is associated with feelings of belonging, significance, connection, growth, certainty, contribution, and so on, so use the term "member" as much as possible, in every conversation, in every advertisement, in every message, on every platform, and so on.

The key to health-club marketing and sales is to find the win-win balance of giving prospects enough value to get them in the door without giving them too much value relative to their investment. But how much is enough and not too much? I knew the only way I was going to find the answer to that question was through experience (trial and error) and more research.

To be successful in marketing and sales, I had to learn the negative and positive emotions prospects associated with health and fitness and joining a health club. Then, I needed to find ways to replace the negative associations with positive associations. For example, I needed to exchange fear with excitement, frustration with growth, worry with security, regret with connection, embarrassment with contribution, hopelessness with significance, and so on. I knew this process could start with the proper ad copy and design. My goal was to get prospects to link positive emotions to my clients' products, no matter what their reputations in the marketplace had been, good or bad. My campaigns needed to raise immediate cash and long-term revenue, but they also needed to build the club's brand within the community.

Let's take a moment now to discuss what other kinds of studies have been done on behalf of MMC® for the health-and-fitness industry. Focus groups are one of the top ways to determine whether a product, service, business concept, and so on is appealing to the public and why or why not. We also gathered valuable feedback via detailed questionnaires to help build a profile of the ideal prospect. We were able to discern what consumers liked or disliked about every microscopic detail of health and fitness products and services. This data gave me a wealth of information to start building the foundation for MMC®.

Observation studies also were incorporated into our research to help identify how consumers viewed health-club memberships. I did the studies in a one-on-one relaxed setting, and they produced valuable insights into the thoughts of potential members and customers. Mall interception with shoppers, and personal interviews conducted in homes were also used to gather relevant information to help with the deconditioned consumer profile. Research is about asking consumers how they feel about products and services. During our interviews, my team and I uncovered important attitudes, perceptions, beliefs, and behaviors that proved invaluable when it came to building the profile.

Massive databases allow marketers such as MMC® to access critical information such as credit-card spending patterns, consumers' purchase habits, and demographic data that enables us to target the preferred demographics. Capturing customer information like this ensures business growth and prevents wasteful spending. This approach allows us to allocate marketing dollars more effectively. We are in an era of exploding information, and I was determined to put CTC and later MMC® at the forefront of the health-club industry when it came to acquiring new members using up-to-date data. Of course, being able to gather all this information via the Internet came much, much later for me and MMC®, but I would be remiss if I did not share this information with you in this book.

If you have the time or labor available, a lot of research information can be found absolutely free. A lot of local and federal institutions conduct research and surveys every minute of the day, most of which can be found on the Internet. Just enter in your search words and phrases into any search engine, and you'll be on your way. Another great source is trade publications and organizations, but remember they too are in business to make money, so do your homework. Don't forget about your local library as another great resource. They have entire sections devoted to research (that may not be found in electronic formats) and provide staff to assist you in finding things fast. Some of these surveys are conducted through the Internet, over the telephone, through snail mail, personal interviews, and so on, but no matter how, when, or why the information was gathered, it will serve as a valuable resource throughout your career.

Some of the things I had hoped to achieve from my research were, becoming aware of perceptions of the health clubs within a given market and learning the likes and dislikes of past, current, and potential members. I wanted to hear suggestions and ideas that could enhance services and products, as well as listen to stories, good and bad, about people's experiences with health clubs. I wanted to uncover patterns of behavior, learn about decision processes, and find out who was involved in the decision processes: spouses, family members, and friends. Most of all, I wanted to learn how to identify and engage the deconditioned market.

Profiling gives you a much greater chance of knowing where and how to focus your marketing efforts, therefore avoiding wasteful spending while increasing profit margins. With this information, I would be able to implement customer-penetration programs, bringing in new business from an untapped segment of the market.

I relied on both qualitative and quantitative studies to profile the targeted market. Qualitative studies include focus groups, mini–focus groups, dyads, triads, in-depth personal interviews, observational studies, and brainstorming sessions, to name just a few. Quantitative studies include segmentation studies, communication studies, advertising-execution studies, advertising-awareness and tracking studies, price studies, and customer-satisfaction research.

My team and I also wanted to understand both strategic research, which helped to determine the most promising and profitable courses of action, and tactical strategies, which helped to determine how best to achieve the courses of action deemed to be most promising as they pertained to the structure of my marketing campaigns.

Now that I had a detailed profile of my target and knew the message I wanted to convey, it was time to find the best form of marketing, advertising, or promotional materials and media to use to engage the profiled targets. I did a ton of research on this subject such as well—communication studies, advertising-execution studies, advertising-awareness and tracking studies, packaging studies were all part of the research that lead me eventually to settle on direct mail as the driving force of my campaigns. I realize this seems overwhelming, and quite frankly, it is. When I first started this journey, I had no idea of the amount of information, education, and data that was needed to successfully penetrate an untapped market.

When I was twenty, I took a few business classes at a community college to have access to professors, but I was not going to obtain the relevant knowledge I needed by attending an institution of higher learning. I didn't have four years to devote to a degree; I had to get back to work, so I needed to stay focused on just the relevant material. I am a true believer in a college education. I understand by attending college you receive a well-rounded education, but I wasn't interested in 90 percent of the curriculum. I wanted to know psychology as it pertains to consumer behavior and more specifically how it affects buying decisions as well as health-club marketing strategies, but unfortunately, there were no traditional educational institutions offering this kind of program.

I had once read you could get the equivalence of a college education driving in your car listening to cassette tapes (this was pre–flash drives) within five years. Up to that point, I had been reading a couple of books per week, I had attended countless seminars and workshops and watched who knows how many VHS tapes, and all I ever listened to in my car were educational cassette tapes. I immersed myself in the material pertinent to achieving results in the specific field of locking up relationships with the deconditioned market. Choosing this educational path kept me from wasting precious time studying subjects that were unlikely to get me to my end goal.

I was determined to design a campaign with a customer-penetration strategy that could not fail, and I was willing to study anything and everything possible to accomplish this goal. Today, MMC®'s research center constantly monitors digital conversations via blogs, chat rooms, e-mails, and social networks like Facebook, Myspace, LinkedIn, and Twitter, where customers are talking about the health-club industry. These digital conversations contain real-time pertinent information for acquiring desirable targets. This is just one way MMC® has grown over the years helping our clients develop a competitive advantage in their markets. But again, when I started out, resources like these were not available.

I was also aware that I must discover the very best delivery system for my message, so I studied: PR; packaging design, direct mail, website content development, e-marketing, radio, television, and so on. Don't be naïve; marketing and advertising are necessary to increase the level of awareness in your community, and if you want to grow your business, you better study all available resources.

In MMC®'s infancy, there were no free platforms like websites, social media, and e-marketing. These new platforms needed to be studied as they hit the marketplace and started grabbing traction. Although I am not a tech guy by any stretch of the imagination, I learned a long time ago to "hire for the position." I hire people who not only were qualified for the job but also loved the job they were being hired to do. As marketing started becoming more

successful in the digital world, I assembled a team of IT professionals to maximize MMC®'s proficiency in the electronic world. But
in the beginning of my career, I had to learn how to maximize the
ROI from traditional media like radio, newspaper, direct mail, and
television ads; these were the four staples when it came to getting
your message out. There are far more resources readily available
to you in 2016 than there were in the late 1980s and 1990s when
I first started this research, so get off your couch, and get started.

The only way to learn the most effective media is through trial
and error. I was and still am very fortunate in this area because
I work with numerous clients in every geographical area imagin-
able and have the flexibility to test new ideas at will because I am
bringing in a ton of revenue; most clubs and even fewer marketers
have this luxury. As I said earlier, different media target different
demographics. For example, if I am targeting the hero generation
and some of the baby boomers, we might focus on newspaper or
radio. If we are targeting generation X as well as baby boomers,
we might focus on direct mail along with some e-marketing and
radio. If we are targeting millennials, we will focus on social media, e-marketing, and SMS as well as direct mail. But if we have the
money, we will always use direct mail as the driving force of the
campaign because hands down it yields the greatest ROI. I always
say we *may* focus on a certain media, but this is not a set rule. Every
project is completely unique, and you must do your research on
a case-by-case basis before launching the campaign, because the
bottom line—is the bottom line.

Back in the day, everyone wanted to run television ads, but TV
commercials are really feasible only for owners of multiple clubs.
When you are running a single health club, commercials are probably one of the worst investments for growing your health club
due to the wide geographical area television serves. On the other
hand, because the reach is so wide and vast, if you have multiple
locations, it can yield a decent return. Of course, this is only if you

have the money to run multiple commercials to make the imprint necessary to get your brand fixed in the viewers' minds, which demands repetitive ads and even more repetition to get viewers to take action. TV commercials have the ability to capture the complete attention of your prospect because you can be creative in your ads through images and sound, which are two very important senses. Television stations have real-time tracking abilities when it comes to knowing the number of people watching at any given time as well as a rudimentary demographic profile of the viewers. The downside to television advertisement is the creative, production, and airtime costs that make it very expensive, in addition to maintaining scripts, concepts, and designs which can be even more expensive, because they all must be rewritten or updated often. Television ads are very short, which requires your ads to be creative enough to get the interest of the audience in just a few seconds and also means you are very limited in your message. Studies also show that in a lot of cases, people do not believe ads they see on TV. Other challenges are customers tend to do something else during commercial breaks, and most importantly, viewers lack station loyalty, which may require you to advertise on more than one station to get the desired result.

Radio is still (as of 2016) a reliable source of getting the message out, especially for generational marketing, although the demographic profile is also elementary at best. The key to this media is you must make sure you can convey your message with a call-to-action in a thirty- or sixty-second spot. Radio engages the auditory senses, so maximize that aspect of your message by being creative with sounds and music. As I discussed earlier, you must get the customers' senses involved, and radio is a great way to achieve this goal. Think about the mood you are looking to set, and then get music that will move your listeners toward that mood. Radio is still a good support media for a marketing campaign because it is cost effective and easy to produce. There are a few negatives, like the geographical area it covers, which probably goes far beyond your business' reach. Yes, 1, 2, or 3 percent of the club's members will come from outside your target market, but their numbers are very low relative to the overall pool of prospects. So, targeting a larger market in most cases is a waste of money, but with radio being so affordable in most markets, I am able to reach enough prospects within the target market to justify the enlarged market reach of the station.

Some of the negatives you hear about radio advertisement are the following: short exposure due to thirty- or sixty-second spots, so just like television, you must do repetitive ads so you'll stick in the listeners' minds; limited time equates to limited content; there is a lack of trackability for ad success rate (although I disagree with this—we at MMC® teach our client's staff to ask every prospect how he or she heard about the club); there is a lack of visual perception from the audience, which makes it hard to remember because the prospect cannot go back to review important details (this is why I couple radio with some print ads); in some cases, radio is considered background noise and does not have a focused audience; ads are sometimes considered to be an unwelcomed interruption of the music, and listeners often switch stations to avoid listening to advertisements; there is no tangible reference for residual effect; radio is notorious for ad clutter (one ad after another); and you must advertise on more than one station simultaneously to reach different demographics. Bottom line, I am a fan of radio despite its negatives but, again, only as a support media and only when I am targeting a specific demographic.

Another media I use to deliver my message is print ads. I do often use them when targeting specific demographic groups with an emphasis on certain generations. With print ads, you can say a lot in a small space. A picture can speak a thousand words, and this is even more true when it comes to print ads. I am a fan of advertising in newspapers (although the core audience is dying off) especially when the ad space can be bartered out. Whether you pay for the ads or barter for them, always make sure you get online ads to support your marketing campaigns. Newspapers allow you to reach a large number of people in a given geographical area, and subscribers are normally loyal customers. When I was a kid growing up in Chicago, my dad had me buy a *Chicago Sun-Times* every Sunday morning from the corner paper box. If I ever got the wrong paper, like the *Tribune*, he would be livid. But again, you must know the demographic you are trying to reach. Older generations are more likely to read the newspaper as a habit, whereas millennials tend to get their news from online platforms.

In Chicago back in the early 1970s, the working class preferred the *Sun-Times*, and the affluent preferred the *Tribune*. You could also go as far as saying the Democrats read the *Times* and the Republicans read the *Tribune* (or the liberals preferred the *Sun-Times*, and the conservatives, the *Tribune*) supporting my theory that large corporations know their targeted audiences. In my younger years, I heard if you're in your twenties and are not a Democrat, you have no heart. If you're in your forties and are not a Republican, you have no money. I don't care either way. My reason for mentioning politics at all is only to open your eyes to profiling a specific demographic or segment of the market and knowing the audience.

Another advantage of advertising in newspapers is the different ad sizes available. This allows you to advertise within your budget. Advertisers will tell you, people have also been known to keep and read newspapers for a few days as well as share them with others, which increases your visibility, although in reality, newspapers are more than likely read once or twice on average. The key to success is to make your ads stand out from the clutter of other ads on a page. Try to place your ads in the top-right corner of the right page; this is the place where your readers will be most likely to notice your ad. Newspaper ads can be expensive since multiple insertions are necessary to make an impact, so do your homework. The biggest downside of newspaper ads is that the demographic they reach is primarily the older generations, and with the explosion of the Internet, there has been a huge decline in newspaper readership.

Direct mail is my preference above all other media. When I first started selling clubs on my Cash campaign, I ran into continuous pushback because of the cost, but I understood the cost was the only true negative for direct mail. If managed properly, direct mail can actually be self-funding. It is imperative to partner with a vendor who is up to date on the latest requirements of the postal service, so the mailing house can do all of the presorting and handling of the mail to get the very best postal rates and preferred times of delivery for clients.

I studied all forms of media but could not get any one of them to perform as well as profiled, personalized direct mail. Direct mail is highly selective and specifically targets the desired market; it allows me to be creative through visual aids; it lands in the hands of 99.9 percent of the prospects on my mailing list; it yields the highest ROI; I can include unlimited content relative to the size of the piece; it is very easy to track the audience's responses; it is cost effective relative to the ROI; it's tangible; it involves essential sensory participation from a person; and most importantly, it allows clients to build an enormous in-house databases for future campaigns. There is only one challenge with direct mail, and that is cost. That is why I had to design my campaigns to be completely (100 percent) self-funding from the very beginning.

If you are a marketer, you must reverse any risk to the customer and sell the result of the product or service. So, when trying to acquire clients, you must show them there is zero downside and that the result will solve at least one of—but hopefully most of—their problems. I am a staunch believer in direct mail (if done correctly) because of the immediate and long-term residual effects a business receives, including but not limited to branding and sales revenue.

Businesspeople want to know the ROI, or the return they'll receive on their marketing dollars. I live, eat, and breathe marketing and sales, so I have a more aggressive attitude to monies spent on marketing than most, but any businessperson knows numbers, and numbers never lie. I think if you are getting an ROI of 10 percent or better, you should keep doing what you are doing, because you're extremely lucky to get that rate of return from any investment. I have frequently seen ROIs from MMC®'s direct-mail campaigns yield 100 to 500 percent; for MMC®, a 100 percent ROI is on the low side. You'll only get that kind of return once in a lifetime, if then, from any other legitimate investment.

It baffles me when owners complain about the cost of direct mail when they are getting a 100 or even 200 percent return. If they just thought of their other investments—such as stocks, bonds, and CDs, which get 3 to 15 percent—they might gain a little perspective. Traditional investments take years to see returns, and with direct mail, the return is immediate as well as long-term. There is absolutely no better investment in business. Besides, I'll invest in my own capabilities before I turn my money over to some fund manager who gets paid win or lose.

Direct mail has numerous advantages over all other media. As I stated earlier, with direct mail, you can write an article, a book, or as much as you want. Although you always want to keep your ad copy short and sweet. You could also put an insert into your direct-mail piece that gives more detailed information, such as a DVD or a flash drive. With direct mail, you are reaching the most qualified prospects available in your target market. You must consider your geographic target market, which is a one-, three-, four-, seven-mile or whatever mile radius is up to a twenty-mile radius around your health club, depending on the drive time. Direct-mail campaigns are sniper campaigns, with each individual qualified prospect in your cross hairs.

When you enlist direct mail as the driving force of your marketing strategy, you can target people through a profiled mailing list using demographic and psychographic data that will help you eliminate wasteful spending and yield a higher ROI. Direct mail is absolutely the best delivery system to capture and acquire the most qualified prospective members—those consumers within your geographical reach that have disposable income.

Since you have no limit on content other than the size of your piece, you can convey a detailed message. It is easy to track your audience's responses effectively with direct mail; costs are controlled by you and your budget, you have full control over creativity and execution from start to stamp, and every piece is personalized and addressed to its recipient (at least, that is how MMC® does direct mail). Direct mail is the most engaging of all advertising, and the impact of direct mail goes far beyond its immediate returns. Direct mail's residual effect brings customers in for months and years to come. It is very hard for your competitors to track and copy your direct mail until you release the mail, which makes copying your pieces a losing proposition.

When it comes to direct mail, volume speaks volumes. Direct mail should be deployed in volume. You must target every "qualified" prospect in your market and get your club in front of them often. Business is a numbers game, and direct mail is a numbers game.

Every owner wants to get the biggest bang for his or her buck from marketing. Direct mail does just that; not only is it a huge revenue producer when it's designed correctly, but it also gives clubs enormous exposure in the right places, which is in their immediate areas. Health-club exposure is just one of the reasons why I choose to use direct mail as the driving force of our campaign. Direct mail also gives health clubs the most exposure from the least investment.

Health-club marketing exposure means you get your brand in front of as many prospective members as possible. This can be done effectively only through direct mail. Most owners have a difficult time understanding the ROI when it comes to direct mail. Direct mail not only gives you the greatest immediate results but also provides the business with long-term residual dividends paid through brand recognition and future sales.

Incorporating behavioral-profiled demographics and direct mail focused on a specific geographical target area puts you in complete control of whom you choose to engage or not engage as a potential customer. No other media offers this in-depth customization as to where exactly your prospects are being harvested and who is being engaged. Some media provide elementary demographic profiles of their customers but are delivered to markets far beyond a client's reach. Some media provide a more desirable geographical market but lack the in-depth profiling needed for your business and your ROI. To give you a better visual, think of radio, television, Internet, newspaper, social media, and most other media as shotguns that fire shells full of hundreds of small pellets, which scatter as soon as they leave the barrel of the gun, hitting anything and everything. Now, imagine a highly qualified sniper in possession of a precision rifle, which has a scope with a range of up to ten miles, locking in on his or her target and squeezing the trigger. There is no wasted investment and definitely no unwanted collateral damage (undesirables). Simply put, all other media are like hunting with a shotgun, and direct mail is like hunting with a precision sniper rifle.

Another reason I love direct mail is that it allows you to repeat the message over and over to pique the prospect's interest, and by doing so, it will start to condition prospects to think of your health club when they think of health and fitness. The only thing better than direct mail would be to go to each "qualified" house in your radius, knock on the door, and introduce your health club with a

PowerPoint presentation. But even then, you would still need the pertinent data to profile qualified prospects, or you would just be wasting 80 percent of your time and money knocking on unqualified doors. There is no better marketing strategy available when it comes to profiling your deconditioned and health-and-fitness-conscious prospects through demographics and psychographics than that of purchasing or renting quality lists based on the prospects' buying patterns and spending habits as well as their geographic locations relative to the health club.

Don't waste marketing dollars on undesirable targets; put your message in the hands of prospective members you would be proud to call members and loyal customers. The power of a personalized offer that is tangible cannot be underestimated. The immediate and residual measurable dividends that a properly executed direct-mail campaign produces are far superior to those from any other form of marketing. Eventually, you want your health club's name in every qualified consumer's mind within your radius. Direct mail is the best delivery system to make that happen; all other media and platforms should be considered support systems and not the driving forces of a full-blown marketing campaign.

Coupons can also be inserted into your direct-mail piece, although some health club owners don't like to use coupons because they think coupons cheapen or devalue their brand. This is not the case at all if they're used properly. The key to using coupons is to be sure you are not diminishing the perceived value of your products and services. Coupons are a great resource to get members in the door when you are looking at marketing options. When looking at all the different social types of members, keep in mind that some groups love coupons, so if you are going to target them (even if you don't want to target anybody looking for coupon deals), you must have this arrow in your marketing quiver. You do not have the luxury of picking and choosing which media your demographic is going to respond to, so you better know how to enlist them all. The key is to design a coupon-marketing campaign that is perceived as offering enormous savings, which is very attractive to the prospective member, yet does not devalue the brand or take away from the bottom line of the business. Think outside the box, and you will discover great ways to use coupons in your marketing strategy.

Although mobile, social, and digital marketing are all effective platforms and are easily measured and tracked, they were not viable candidates in the early stages of CTC and then later for MMC®. It wasn't until the past few years when they were considered mainstream media. As I stated earlier, I believe all media have their good and bad points, and I am a firm believer in all formats and platforms. Today, MMC® employs a team of experts in social media and e-marketing, but I still find these media and platforms lacking in some areas. Millennials make up the largest percentage of consumers for social media, SMS, and e-marketing. But even today, direct mail hands down produces the best overall results.

Almost all health clubs are basically the same on the surface; athletic clubs, fitness centers, gyms, and so on are essentially all selling the use of weights, group classes, and cardio equipment. But you can catapult yourself over your competitors if you bring in the differential advantages of your club: the work-out experience, your swimming pool, Jacuzzi, the spa, the pro shop, the tanning salon, and so on. As a health-club marketer, I have to identify and highlight what differential advantages my clients have over their competitors and capitalize on those features, advantages and benefits. Every health club has its own advantages; it is your job to identify and highlight yours. This may be your unique selling proposition or some advantage your health club has through its operations, such as a line of equipment or the service it provides. It just takes a little time and research to determine your differential advantage over your competitor, and there could be numerous advantages.

Marketing a health club means discovering what advantages a member will receive by joining your loyalty program as opposed to your competitor's: find out what separates you from your competitor, what makes your health club's rates a better value than your competitor's, and so on. Start learning by asking yourself good questions, and your brain will give you great answers. These are the same questions members are asking themselves: Which is better, health club ABC or health club XYZ? Why should I join ABC health club over XYZ health club? These questions are going through prospects' minds, and you must have those answers readily available. Put those answers out in the front for your community to see.

Price analysis plays a very important role in health-club marketing, but most health clubs fail to conduct this analysis properly. Most health clubs are raising their membership fees but have no solid research or increased value to substantiate or justify the increase. What I did when I was conducting research was go out into the marketplace and expose the true value as well as the perceived value of my clients' health clubs, because it doesn't really matter what the owners think the value of the membership is; the only thing that really matters is what the market thinks. In my research, I had to identify how much the prospective member was willing to pay before I put a price for a membership out into the marketplace. The market may not have the same perceived value of your products and services as you do. Your perceived value is irrelevant to the paying member, who will dictate your pricing structure, or at least a portion of it, whether you like it or not. Far too often, clubs price their memberships based on their competitors' rates. This is absurd. But the absurdity doesn't stop there. Some clubs price their memberships out of the market, and others price their memberships too low—devaluing their own product.

You can't just set your rates for memberships without conducting some fundamental research. You have to look at the market and discover what your health club can command. Failing to analyze your pricing structure is business suicide. Ascertain how much other health clubs with similar facilities are charging their members. Notice what the health-and-fitness market is willing to pay. Then, determine where your club fits into the picture based on your amenities, niche(s) and services, and then determine your rates based on your research and not your competitors. All of these questions can be answered by doing an in-depth competitive overview before settling on a price-point. Focus on the competitors within a twenty-mile radius of your club. This is as far as you'll ever pull the majority of your members from, so don't waste your money or time outside of this radius.

As I was conducting my initial research, I also needed to discover a universal price-point, which meant I had to go far beyond the local market and look at prices from a national viewpoint. I had to analyze the pricing of twenty thousand health clubs across the United States, uncover a national average, and divide the average member's usage by that price to determine the average daily visit price. Then, I multiplied that number by the number of visits recorded by deconditioned consumers to introduce a realistic number that could be used as a hook to grab the attention of this difficult-to-reach segment. Once I had that number, I had to test numerous number combinations to determine which numbers were going to have the biggest draw. This formula didn't come to me overnight. It took a while, but it was worth the time, money, and effort. You need to create your own formula when settling on your pricing structure.

I also tested all different types of introductory memberships as packages that would complement the hooks to get people through the door without giving the club away, including daytime memberships, every-other-day memberships, limited-hour memberships, buy-one-get-one-free memberships, pay-as-you-go memberships, monthly dues memberships, and countless others before ever unearthing the perfect membership package to offer. In chapter 7, I'll go into the details of MMC®'s famous Cash campaign and walk you through the process of how all of this research and the data it provided me formed the membership that revolutionized the health-club industry.

CHAPTER 7

THE MEMBERSHIP THAT REVOLUTIONIZED THE HEALTH-CLUB INDUSTRY

After profiling and then surveying the deconditioned segment, my team found that 90 percent of the interviewees said cost, customer service, and convenience were their deciding factors when choosing a health club, whereas only 10 percent attributed their decisions to amenities and facilities. This is the polar opposite of the health-and-fitness-conscious population, of whom 90 percent said amenities and facilities contributed to their buying decisions. Part of the story told by our studies is that 90 percent of customers surveyed who fell in the uncommitted category said they would be more likely to join if prices were lower, customer service was better, and the location was more convenient. I listened to the public and designed MMC®'s Cash campaign around the consumers' unmet needs, wants, wishes, and desires, all the while making sure we did not discount the membership or devaluing the product.

All of this data proved I was on the right track. My entire career thus far was built on the theory that if I could just lower the barrier-to-entry, focus on volume, focus external marketing on the uncommitted segments, and focus internal marketing on promoting the profit centers, I could increase sales (revenue) tenfold. The key to a successful campaign is to do the complete opposite of what all the industry's "experts" preach. The industry "experts" brainwash owners into thinking they can charge exorbitant fees, including initiation fees or enrollment fees, and then forget about the members, who were locked into one or two-year agreements. I saw numerous flaws in this model over the years, including the obvious, that it alienated a huge portion of the market and led to poor renewal (retention) rates.

Everyone in the industry is thinking short-term. There are numerous studies done on how much it costs to acquire a new customer (member) as opposed to retain an existing one. The average cost to acquire a new member works out to be approximately six times more than it does to retain an existing member. In short, you save six times the revenue by servicing and then renewing your members than by replacing your members. This is far from a revelation for most savvy businesspeople, although it may be for others, but even those who know this fact fail to understand it in relative terms. This number must then be added to the lifetime value of the member, not just the up-front revenue or the one-year membership contractual number, to realize the true value of the member.

Once you know the value of your member, you will know how much you can afford to spend to acquire a new member as well as how much you'll earn per member. There are some health-club owners who are reluctant to try MMC®'s Cash campaign because they look at the hook (price-point) only as a one-and-done without any additional fees; they are simply unaware of the true value of each member and the massive back-end revenue contributed to these elusive consumers. Owners know they need new memberships to continue the operations of the club, but they don't realize the impact a single new member has on the bottom line for years to come.

I want owners to start thinking about long-term revenue as opposed to what they need today. Each prospective member has a value; let's use X as that value and multiply it by how many prospective members we can attract through a single marketing campaign. This is exactly what I did: the X amount (revenue raised) determined how much my clients could afford to spend on each campaign. I was focusing on the bottom line: how many new members the marketing campaign would attract, how much immediate and residual revenue the campaign was going to raise, and so on. Then, I worked my way back through the numbers to determine how much money the club was going to invest (but first I would raise the money) into my Cash campaign to acquire each new member. After that, it was simple math to determine whether it was a good investment.

Another important aspect of knowing the real value of each prospective member is once you know the dollar value of each prospect, you tend to work harder on cultivating each relationship because you know the true value of the prospect is not just $30 (or whatever your monthly dues are) but could end up being $5,000 to $10,000 in future revenue.

I needed a way to lower the barrier-to-entry enough to attract the masses so I could increase traffic and increase daily receivables through profit-center revenue, which in turn would offset or even surpass the revenue owners imagined they would lose. In short, I wanted to redistribute the revenue stream. I first thought of this from an experience I had when I was fifteen (in 1978). I was staying with my aunt and uncle in Chicago for a couple of months; they lived on Southport and Irving Park on the North Side, just a few blocks from Wrigley Field. One night, my cousins informed me we would be driving out to the suburbs the following day. Everyone was excited because we were going to a store called Walmart; I didn't share their enthusiasm, because I had worked all week in a warehouse, and the weekend was supposed to be for fun, not for driving a couple of hours through city traffic, crammed in the back seat of a tiny Ford Falcon, just to go shopping, when we had at least four grocery stores within ten blocks of their house.

Once we arrived at Walmart, I immediately understood why everyone was so excited. First, the parking lot was packed. Cars were everywhere, and everyone I saw was smiling and happy. You could literally see how excited everyone was to be there. People were scurrying through the parking lot to get through the store entrance; some were dressed to the hilt, some not so well, but most were just everyday hardworking people like my aunt and uncle. As we entered through the doors, everything was bright and beautiful. There were more products than I had ever seen in a single store. Kids were staring at toys with their mouths open wide in disbelief. Teenage boys and girls were playing with balls, bicycles, and electronics. Moms were looking through household products and clothing; dads were in the lawn-and-garden section. There was literally something for everyone. We all had a fantastic time shopping at Walmart that day, and the entire family went home with something.

I believe that was on a Saturday, because the following day, my uncle and I were sitting out on the front porch, people-watching and talking. I told him how cool Walmart was and how much I had really enjoyed going there and thanked him for taking me. But even back then, I was very inquisitive. I was one of those precocious kids you call a pain in the behind when they are growing up but then geniuses when they're older and successful. Like most kids, I had Teflon skin and didn't care whether people thought I was a pain in the behind or not; I was just being inquisitive. I asked my uncle why he drove all the way out there to shop when we lived in the middle of countless stores. His answer was really simple: "Because at Walmart, I can afford to buy a little something for everyone, and it's all under one roof." Now, that was genius!

From then on, I studied models like Walmart and Sam's club as well as their founder, Sam Walton. His philosophy was to serve the everyday consumer—the masses—and make his company's money on volume and variety. I once read if you want to earn more money, give more value; if you want to earn even more money, give even more value. Sam Walton knew this and implemented it on a mass scale. He knew the elite class was very small (less than 20 percent of the population), disloyal, and extremely difficult to penetrate, whereas the average everyday consumer, comprising 80 percent of the population, was not only penetrable but far more loyal. This is a very simple concept, yet some industry guys can't grasp it and still focus on the membership cost and not the enormous overall residual income that can be earned from thousands of happy, loyal members.

I knew the first challenge was to find the magic number for the introductory membership that would be so good no one could pass it up—basically I wanted to make everyone an offer they couldn't refuse—but at the same time, it needed to be a number that could be universally successful in any geographical area. There have been numerous studies on number combinations and how they are received by consumers. Do I use a four-digit number, a three-digit number, or a two-digit number? Should it end with an eight, a nine, a zero, and so on? These studies helped a lot with the academics of the campaign and provided the pertinent data, but the only way I would ever know the answers to all of my questions as well as the validity of my theories was by testing several combinations in the real world, and my answer would lie in the results.

There is a marketing reality called the pique technique. The pique technique teaches you to stay away from the norm when advertising. Human brains are lazy and take millions of shortcuts when processing things we see in an attempt to conserve energy. If our eyes see something familiar, our brains tend to scan over it because they assume they already know what is coming next. If you want your advertising to get noticed, the worst thing you can do is repeat the same offer over and over again (including repeating your competitors' offers). You have to change it up, or the consumer will soon be immune to it.

I knew ninety-nine dollars had worked extremely well as a hook in the past because that was the number we used in the promotion companies I had worked with before, but by the late 1980s and early 1990s, a lot of health clubs were copying and abusing the ninety-nine-dollar hook, and consumers were seeing it everywhere. Now, I was seeing it everywhere from aerobics-only memberships to initiation fees, summer memberships to full unlimited one-year memberships. That is still one of the biggest problems that plague the health-club industry today—copycats. Club owners and managers see their competitors run a promotion, and without any research or education, they try to copy it immediately. These clueless geniuses don't realize they know only what their competitors, or whoever has designed the campaigns, want them to know. These clubs who copy the price-point are getting the same information being blasted to the consumer, and they are taking the bait just like the consumer.

Think of launching a marketing campaign like MMC®'s Cash campaign to going fishing; before ever baiting a hook, you must have a plan. The night before, as you prepare for the event, you decide what species you want to fish for (demographic); which location you'll fish (geographical area); what bait you'll fish with (offer); the habits of the species of fish you are targeting (lifestyles); the depth you'll fish (what days and times you want your marketing to hit the public for the fullest impact); whether you need to bring additional equipment, such as bobbers, different-size hooks, lures, and so on (supplemental media); whether you're fishing all day or overnight (duration); and what the migration habits of the fish are (how you keep your current members in place and how to prevent them from migrating to the new offer), as well as a thousand other questions that must be answered before you even leave the house. You don't just say, "OK, I have the hook and a worm; now, let me go compete with the pro anglers." Yet people somehow hypnotize themselves and others into believing they know how to run their neighbors' campaigns.

I have come to understand this phenomenon of taking the path of least resistance well as I study the industry. I put people who chose to rely on their competitor's for new ideas into two classifications—the too busy and the morally challenged. The too-busy person busts his or her butt all day, wearing more hats than a hat rack can hold. This person does every task in the club. Whether this onslaught has been self-imposed or assigned, either way, it is a recipe for overload, mismanagement, and inevitable burnout. The morally challenged on the other hand, are so afraid of losing their jobs or being failures, they spend more time in fear than on innovation. People like this are always looking for the shortcut—the easy way. I am not going to say there are no shortcuts in life, because there is at least one. It's called accelerated learning, and if you use it wisely, the knowledge you acquired can be used to catapult you far beyond your competitors. But you must know when a shortcut is a shortcut and not a path that leads you over a cliff. It is these unscrupulous individuals who have put the health-club industry into the mess it is in today.

The majority of owners of health clubs normally get into the business because they are health-and-fitness fanatics. They live, eat, and breathe health and fitness just as I live, eat, and breathe marketing and professional sales. They come into the industry for the right reasons—to provide a valuable service for an honest return. People go into business to serve others and make livings. Unfortunately, a lot of the morally challenged have made it extremely difficult to earn a good living in the health-club business today. These morally challenged have skimmed the top off the business to the point that every health-club owner in America must work ten times harder just to get by. I have never seen times as difficult as they are today in this business, and it is absolutely avoidable, especially when you read the data on the percentage of Americans interested in diet and exercise. Later, in the final chapter, I will lay out a detailed plan to get the industry back to its glory days, but right now, I'm getting ahead of myself, so back to the membership that revolutionized the industry.

The ninety-nine-dollar offer was a huge draw, but like everything, when the newness wore off, the response will drop off as well. So, I needed to make a new twist on an old hook. Always remember it's a waste of time to try to reinvent the wheel. Just complement the original design by making it better, faster, cooler, smoother, and so on which is completely different than copying. The wheel is the wheel but you can compare the wheel off a horse and buggy from the 1800s next to a one-off rim from a custom 2016 Escalade, and although both of them are wheels, there is a world of difference between them. A health-club membership is a health-club membership and there is no reason to change the product, but the price-point, packaging, and presentation of the membership are only hooks, and a hook needs to be changed.

I really liked the response from the ninety-nine-dollar hook, and since the amount collected at the point of sale played a major role in making the campaign successful and self-funding, it was a perfect place to start. You must collect enough money up-front to pay for the expenses of the campaign, and you must also be able to show the owner an immediate ROI, or he or she will never agree to do the campaign. But as I said, I couldn't use ninety-nine dollars as the hook, because everyone in the business was using it every day and killing its effectiveness. I could only use it as a frame of reference to design the new hook.

The challenge with any type of hook like this is selling club owners on the idea. Most owners are not marketers or salespeople. It is very difficult for them to think far enough outside the box to understand that the price is just a marketing hook to grab prospects' attention. Owners get their information from industry magazines, their competitors, or other owners and industry people. Unfortunately, sometimes when it comes to growing a health club or a business, it is the blind leading the blind, especially when it comes to marketing and sales. When owners hear a hook like the $99, they automatically think it's too cheap and the price-point will ruin their businesses, because again, all they see is the price-point and not the overall revenue. They "assume" the program is a fire-sale (due to past experiences with previous unscrupulous promoters) designed to get a bunch of cash up-front and to hell with tomorrow. From the inception of this new marketing strategy I had to make sure the Cash campaign was going to be engineered to bring in daily receivables, monthly receivables, member loyalty, as well as tons of up-front cash collected at the point of sale.

Club owners tend to focus so intently on monthly receivables that the grim reaper of being cash-poor creeps up and bite them in the butt. Then, and only then, do they change their focus to raising cash, but unfortunately, it is out of desperation instead of forward thinking. They now lose focus on monthly dues and make desperate attempts to raise cash. It has always been a challenge to balance up-front cash with long-term residual revenue. I was determined to rectify all of that by creating a campaign that would not only bring in obscene amounts of cash but also increase daily revenue, as well as monthly receivables. And guess what: I did exactly that.

I had the number I was going to use, and no, it was not ninety-nine dollars. That was no longer the magic number. It had been beaten to death, and everyone knows there is no reason to beat a dead horse. Now I needed to design a membership that was attractive enough to get people to say yes but perfectly balanced between value and investment. I hated those promotions of the past because they were devastating to clubs and devalued the product, which resulted in a loss for everyone but the promotion companies. The owners lost because they had no residual income, and the members lost because the clubs cut back on services or, even worse, eventually went out of business. The industry lost as a whole because health-club memberships were devalued. I had to design a package that left some meat on the bone for future meals. So, I started running more free campaigns for clubs to test different variations of membership packages.

As I discussed briefly in the previous chapters, I tested numerous ideas, such as off-peak hours, special events, summer memberships, two for ones, buy-one-get-one-free offers, and on and on, but none ever worked at the magnitude I needed. All of those campaigns were successful on various levels, but I wasn't looking for mediocre results; I was looking to revolutionize the health-club industry. I finally decided on limiting the days. I knew most health-and-fitness enthusiasts tried to work out every other day— for example, Monday, Wednesday, and Friday—although most members frequently skipped Friday nights because they tended to party if they were living a single's lifestyle or to spend time with their families otherwise. Fewer members chose the Tuesday, Thursday, and Saturday routines, but if they did, they tended to miss Saturdays for similar reasons as the Monday, Wednesday, Friday crowd. I'm not talking about the hard-core gym rats; I'm referring to the overall membership base. I also knew from experience you could shoot a cannon through most health clubs on Fridays, Saturdays, and Sundays without hitting a single member (although that has changed a little in the past decade).

I started off with a weekend membership, and it tanked. Then, I decided I would try a four-day membership that allowed new members to work out on Tuesdays, Thursdays, Saturdays, and Sundays; this membership did much better, but it still didn't produce anywhere near the numbers I needed. So, I tried a new combination and rolled out a four-day membership that gave new members access on Thursdays through Sundays, and the results were relatively the same. I then rolled out a membership consisting of five days

per week—Tuesdays, Thursdays, Fridays, Saturdays, and Sundays—
and the numbers rocked. Wow, the response was fantastic, equal
to or even greater than the numbers of the past promotion companies who had given the entire club away. I was ecstatic with the
results.

I had now discovered the perfect package to blow the roof off,
but this celebration was short-lived as well. My goal was to offer a
limited introductory membership with an option to upgrade to
a full club membership with no restrictions. Unfortunately, this
package failed to deliver on the upgrades. In fact, with this package, only a handful of the new members upgraded. We were no
better off than with the original promotion, other than the club
wasn't any busier on Mondays and Wednesdays, which was good
for traffic distribution, but this was not my only goal. I needed to
generate upgrades and add-ons (up sales) for future revenue to
make this a successful campaign. This so-called success was nothing more than a disaster in my opinion; I was horrified with the
results, to say the least. Anyone else would have thought they had
struck gold, but I knew this campaign would hurt a club long-term,
and I was in it for the long haul.

Another disheartening thing I discovered after interviewing
the new members was a large portion of the new members came
from the health-and-fitness-conscious segment because the days of
the membership were easily adaptable to their schedules. They felt
all they were losing was Monday by the way the new membership
was packaged. In reality that was not at all the case, but perception
is people's reality, and if they perceived the membership that way
then it was that way to them. This was not at all what I wanted to
hear.

I needed to make the membership valid five days a week because the response to my marketing was spot-on. I just needed
to diminish the response from the health-and-fitness-conscious
and augment the response from the deconditioned segment. I

started thinking about the traffic in a health club again and the conditioned way fitness-minded people thought in the 1980s and 1990s. Everyone was conditioned to work out at least three days a week, and normally that was Mondays, Wednesdays, and Fridays or Tuesdays, Thursdays, and Saturdays. Reality (data), however, proved the clubs' traffic diminished as the week came to an end and was almost nonexistent on Saturdays and Sundays. This is why you must study the human psyche as well as data. I decided to go with a Wednesday-through-Sunday membership, eliminating Mondays and Tuesdays from their respective three-day regimens, since these were the two busiest days for clubs, as well as the main days of the two regimens, which would discourage any health-and-fitness-conscious prospects and existing members from joining on the introductory membership.

The campaign was a grand slam. The response rate was awesome; the upgrades from the five-day to the seven-day membership hit almost 30 percent, and migration of existing members to the introductory membership plan were minimal. I had finally done it. I had the perfect membership package, price, and delivery system. The club owner had more cash than he had ever dreamed of; there were over one thousand new members (with the majority coming from an untapped market), which drove up daily revenue in the profit centers by 200 percent from the new traffic on the slower days of the week; the campaign completely paid for itself; this club's name was now in the mind of every qualified resident in the immediate area; and these new members were bringing in friends and relatives, who were joining at the rack rates. Everything was perfect. The Wednesday-through-Sunday membership was the perfect draw and balance of value relative to investment.

I don't want you to think those other membership offers didn't pull an acceptable response, because they did. I even ran a Friday-Saturday-and-Sunday campaign that had a modest return. My challenge was I was not hired for modest returns. When people hire me and MMC®, they want big results fast, and I was designing a campaign that could produce massive results immediately every time. I knew I would only have one-shot at running each campaign because I was not an employee, and if I did not produce extraordinary results, I wouldn't be in business long; there would be no mulligan for MMC®. I also knew my campaign needed to produce consistent results as well. I needed a club in Ashville, North Carolina, to be able to generate the same revenue as a club in Chicago, Illinois, or Los Angeles, California.

When I was on the road selling those old promotions, I would have at least two or three owners a week tell me, "You may have done a hundred thousand dollars in such-and-such club, but you will never do that here. This town (or city, market, or state) is different, these people are different, our economy is different, and, hell, our "dogs" are different. What most people don't understand is numbers are numbers, and business, as well as sales and marketing, are also based on numbers. The offers, amenities, price-point, packaging methods, and so on need to be tailored to each individual club, but the buying habits and spending patterns of the deconditioned and health-and-fitness-conscious segments are the same in every city, town, and state. As long as I had enough of a population that fit my profile within the club's geographical reach, I knew I could get the same or at least similar results every time.

One of the biggest hurdles I had to cross, and still do, was club owners immediately "assume" I am discounting the membership by selling it for a price-point around $99 per year. What they are failing to see is the overall concept of volume pricing and the lifetime value of each member. It is far better to have two thousand members pay you $100 per year than to have five hundred pay $400 per year, and here is why. There are only a finite number of health-and-fitness-conscious consumers within a geographical area willing to commit to a health club by purchasing a membership, and even fewer are willing to pay $400 or more per year for a membership. You must also take into consideration all the other clubs in the area that are competing for those members as well. Remember, research proves amenities are most important to the health-and-fitness-conscious but far less important to the casual user. This means unless you are the top dog in your market, you must be creative with your marketing to make up for what you lack in size, amenities, programs, staff, and so on. The concept is to attract and capture at least a thousand casual users to offset the few hundred heavy users.

Another part of my team's research showed members who spent $400 per year will spend significantly less day-to-day than the members who spent less than one hundred dollars per year. This segment (the casual users) will spend far more in your profit centers; plus, there are hundreds (hopefully thousands) of them now, which increases traffic and therefore drastically increases profit-center revenue. The member who spends more expects more and doesn't expect to pay additional fees or spend additionally on other services, whereas those members who perceive they paid very little in comparison to value are more apt to spend even more than their counterparts, because the spending is never perceived as a large amount of money. So, by having a larger portion of casual users, you will have a greater chance of increasing daily, monthly, and annual revenue.

This reality of casual users spending more in profit centers is completely foreign to most owners because they can only relate to what they know. Owners know when they give discounts on membership rates the club attracts penny-pinching members who can squeeze eleven cents out of every dime. This is because the club is marketing the membership rates to health-conscious consumers— not the deconditioned market. My team sees this all the time. For example, on average health-and-fitness-conscious consumers as a group rarely pay for personal training, whereas the deconditioned consumer as a group ask for help about 80 percent of the time. MMC® profiles, engages and locks up relationships with consumers who have disposable income—not the health-and-fitness-conscious penny-pinchers.

I have always thought health-club memberships should be priced around $360 per year. I am referring to a basic fitness membership—not racquet sports or other niche programs. With that in mind, I knew almost all health clubs had offered a two-for-one or a buy-one-get-one-free membership at one time or another. Since a lot of health clubs offered a seven-day membership for around $360 per year, I decided to base my seven-day upgrade around $360 for two years; basically making it a two for one. Of course, every club is different; some clubs MMC® has worked with charge as much as $600 for a seven-day upgrade during our Cash campaign, some couldn't charge even $100, and others couldn't offer a five-day option at all. This balancing act has been an integral part of the success of the Cash campaign since its inception, and I only learned the perfect balance through trial and error. No two health clubs' businesses are exactly the same, so you just can't assign some arbitrary number to the Cash campaign's introductory offer or the upgrade.

Deciding what to put in and what to leave out of the membership package is also crucial to the success or failure of each campaign. In almost every case, the owner and manager are completely off base when it comes to this part of the campaign. In the initial setup of every health club's campaign, my team and I always consult with the club's owner and manager to get their input because no one knows their day-to-day business as they do. Unfortunately, in most cases, they are way too close to their own product to give unbiased input on what we should offer and at what price-point; their opinions reflect their perceived value, not the reality of the marketplace. Because they have invested so much of their blood, sweat, and tears into the business, and are always dealing with health-and-fitness-conscious consumers, they look at the product with an unrealistic bias. It is too difficult for them to step outside of their cocoon and objectively view the club as the public does, and even deeper—as the casual user does.

I designed the Cash campaign to revolutionize the fitness industry by making health and fitness affordable for all, which meant I would be working with clubs already in existence (or at least that was the case in the beginning). This campaign was not designed for presales and was definitely never meant to be a business model. It was designed to help preexisting clubs capture an elusive segment of the market. Clubs were (and still are) struggling to capture their market share due to supply outpacing demand; for the record, this is the industry's *experts'* opinion, not mine. I know the industry is not overbuilt; it is just inadequately marketed. There is still plenty of business for everyone if the powers that be will just get out of their own way and consider the possibilities of doing something other than what their neighbors are doing. Another obstacle for club owners to get over is to stop listening to the organizations that make their livings off of telling owners what they want to hear.

Albert Einstein defined insanity as doing the same thing over and over again while expecting a different result. Most people (yes, this includes health-club owners) go through the circle of insanity at least once in their business careers. They get to a point where the pain is so great they have to change, so they take action; soon the pain reduces, so they lose their drive or motivation; then, they stop taking action all together and inevitably go right back to where they started. Most of the time, they are even worse off than they were when they started. Now they have to take action again because the pain (motivation) has returned, which causes the vicious cycle of insanity to repeat.

You see this every day with people trying to lose weight. The pain is so great they go on a diet, then they start to lose a little weight, then they start to feel better about themselves, and soon the pain is gone. Before they know it, they are hiding in a closet, eating a slice of cake with a bowl of ice cream. Within six months, they are heavier than ever and full of pain: it's time to start another diet—or, should I say, time to start the cycle of insanity again. Most health clubs are just doing the same old e-mail blasts, newspaper ads, and so on, that they have done for the past one, five, and even ten years, or even worse, they are copying their competitors when they see something they think is new. Doing the same old advertising and promotions year after year is insane.

Students trained in traditional marketing concepts insist the term for my marketing concept is loss-leader marketing (where something is sold at a loss to draw in customers); I strongly disagree and choose to call (and coined) this concept "lost-leader" marketing, because my goal is to get club owners to identify with the concept of looking for resources they already have but have either overlooked or not discovered. "Loss" implies no longer having something, as when something is sold at a loss, whereas "lost" implies something is wasted or not taken advantage of which can be found and used as a resource.

I find the areas of my clients' businesses that have been wasted and not taken advantage of as opposed to making them feel as though they must suffer losses to draw in new customers. It is not my intention to have them sell anything at a loss, nor do I want them to conceptualize this concept as having to lose something to gain something in return—a trade-off. My Cash campaign is built around the concept of finding possible resources that may have been wasted or not taken advantage of—for example, slow times and slow seasons—and maximizing their potential. No client will lose anything; my clients only gain new members, hence the term "lost-leader marketing."

Another one of my objectives for the Cash campaign is to get existing members to remain loyal while prospects give the club a first or second look, which meant I needed to engineer a plan to keep existing members from migrating over to the new introductory membership. I have seen the havoc fire-sale promotions have played on clubs when their core members switch over to a promotional membership. I was never going to let this happen. I was determined to make enough of a difference between my introductory membership and the club's normal membership so all customers (existing members and new prospects alike) could clearly see the difference in value between the two memberships. I designed the program to generate repeat business (long-term revenue) as well as pull in unheard of amounts of cash at the point of sale. I was determined to make it a mathematical improbability (if not an impossibility) that all (or even the majority) of the strong (repeat) relationships of the health club would jump on our offer; my goal was to keep existing members in place with their existing memberships.

With my new introductory membership, I needed to assure club owners they were not giving their clubs away but using the introductory membership only as a hook to fill in slow times and drive revenue into the business during slow seasons, so I decided to use the airline industry as an example. I will expand upon the airline analogy I used earlier in chapter 5. Think of the seating arrangement in a passenger jet. The airline has a great deal invested in safety, equipment, personnel, training, fuel, licenses, computers, software programs, insurance policies, and so on. The airline's plane has an excellent first-class cabin with all of the desired amenities; in addition, they have also developed a business-class cabin for the flyer who desires additional services but can't or won't pay for first-class accommodations. After the airline's first-class and business-class passengers get settled in, the owners looked out over the seating of the airplane and realized over 85 percent of the seats were empty. Now, they still have to pay their pilots, mechanics, flight crews, safety inspectors, fuel costs, and countless other daily expenses, but they just can't get enough bodies in the first-class and business-class seats. They need another seating classification, so they decide to incorporate a coach-class. Coach customers enter their cabin through the same door of the plane, they share the aisle and the air conditioning with business and first-class, and they arrive safely at their destination at the same time as first-class and business-class customers. But, it is certainly not the same travel experience. Less than 5 percent of the plane is occupied by first-class passengers; now add an ambitious 10 percent for business class, which means the plane is comprised of 85 percent coach-class passengers and only 15 percent upper-class. But keep in mind; it is the coach-class customers who make the trip affordable for first- and business-class travelers. If the entire plane were upper-class seating, travelers would pay ten times the amount they pay today, and most airlines would be out of business, because there are nowhere near enough travelers with that kind of disposable income to sustain the business, much less several businesses catering to the same market.

My approach was to design three levels of membership, starting with an entry-level membership (with limited days of use) with a lower barrier-to-entry and all other services (outside of a basic fitness membership) are à la carte. I repeat: this system is not discounting your rates or dues; it is simply redirecting the revenue stream. You collect less up-front but far more over the term of the membership.

Next is a midlevel membership with no limitations on the days of use; the member pays more up-front and also follows the same à la carte system. In most cases, under this membership plan, these members pay as much or even more than the health club is receiving from existing members under its current rate structure.

The final membership is the full, all-inclusive membership you might currently have in place today. This is the membership level everyone will secretly aspire to. These are the members who work out four to five times a week, want to play tennis or racquetball during prime times and reserve the courts well in advance, want people to know their names when they come in the club, want to have their own lockers, want to play in all the club's events, whether tournaments or leagues, don't want to be charged additional fees, want to walk in the club and get immediate attention and recognition, want towel service, want to attend the social functions, and so on. This quality of service, attention, and unlimited access commands a premium membership fee.

To continue with the airline analogy, customers who have flown for many years hate the new airline business model. In the same way, your health-and-fitness-conscious members will hate the new introductory offer and therefore will be unlikely to migrate to the new à la carte membership, feeling they will be nickeled-and-dimed to death. On the other hand, customers who are new to flying and not conditioned to the old flight package love the new à la carte system, perceiving it as paying only for what they use. This will be the same reaction from the deconditioned market that is unfamiliar with the original membership model.

It is difficult to change the preconditioned buying habits of an existing member, whereas it is very easy (with the proper training of your staff) to condition the buying and spending habits of a new member. Unlike the airline industry, I believe existing preconditioned members should be allowed to keep their status quo, while most of the new members acquired from the deconditioned segment are brought in on a new à la carte membership with the option of upgrading to an all-inclusive platinum membership. I knew from years of experience the only way this model would work was if my company (MMC®) tailored the memberships around the clubs' existing business models. There was no way I was going to be able to design a cookie-cutter campaign or a one-size-fits-all type of campaign. Each project would be unique to each health club.

The greatest challenge to this model of drawing in customers with a limited membership was the lack of health-and-fitness-conscious consumers and the damn-near impossible task of reconditioning existing members' habits, both spending and lifestyle. I knew from past trials the core members wanted to work out on Mondays, Tuesdays, and Wednesdays and most notably between 4:00 p.m. and 8:00 p.m. I needed to work around the busy times and bring in members when the club was dead. I would need to design my campaign to target the untapped market that no health club had the resources to identify, engage, or lock up relationships with, and then condition those new members to use the club during slow times and slow seasons.

With this approach to marketing, MMC® could successfully convert fickle price-jumping members into committed, loyal, free-spending members of their new homes. Once a club has a member in a committed relationship, the staff has the time to sell the new member on staying loyal. You can do the same when selling your products or services. The same process I used to design my Cash campaign can be applied to any health-and-fitness product or service—do the research, know your target market, and adjust the pricing and model accordingly. Remember, the hardest thing about the health-club business is getting prospects through the door. Once they are in the club, you need to focus your attention on locking up the relationship. After that, it's all about customer service and retention.

Everything in life is perception (because people's perceptions are their realities). Members must perceive the value of the savings they are receiving as an enormous deal; at the same time, you must make sure you are not tarnishing your brand in the marketplace. This is a delicate balancing act, but it can be accomplished easily with the proper marketing campaigns and experience. Look at your marketing programs, and review what you have to offer: your profit centers, your memberships, and all the different possible revenue resources available. You want to make sure your prospects and community are going to associate nothing but good feelings and positive emotions with your health club. Start thinking of some buzzwords, keywords, or phrases you know are going to resonate with your prospects. Think of your market, think of some of the characteristics you would love to know about a health club if you were in the prospect's shoes. Think of things that would attract you. Think of words that describe emotions that would trigger positive feelings, and incorporate them into your marketing and advertising.

Health-club marketing requires thinking about the value of your brand in terms of its emotional equity: How does it make your prospects and members feel? Once you know how they feel about being members and working out at your club, capitalize on those positive emotions, and convey them in your ad copy and design. There are two questions you must ask yourself before launching a campaign, and then stick the answers into your ad copy. First, can I justify customers buying my products and services now? Second, can I prove to them why they need to buy it now?

One of the early things I learned when studying marketing was the acronym FAB. FAB stands for features, advantages, and benefits. It is extremely important to highlight a product's or service's advantages over its competing products and services, and the benefits derived by the prospect choosing those products or services over their competitors'. Since learning this acronym, I have made it a point to outline the features, advantages, and benefits of all of my clients' clubs, because these FABs (selling points) will make prospects choose my clients' clubs over their competitors' most of the time.

Success doesn't happen by accident; it happens by design. Unless you own an ultraexclusive health club with a waiting list, you should think of your business as a numbers game—the more members, the more revenue. All that should matter when it comes to health-club marketing (other than that it is done with dignity and integrity) is the ROI. The only way I know to sell anything is through ethical principles with the focus on the ROI. I always tell the truth, I always let prospects know what they are receiving in return for their investment.

Marketing and sales go hand in hand, and this is why I never understand how a health club can hire a marketing company to launch a marketing campaign if the owner of the marketing company doesn't have a sales background. Marketing is selling to the masses; if you can't sell or don't know how to sell health-club memberships to individuals, how on earth can you sell to the masses? Even worse, the marketing company cannot train the club's staff on the fundamentals of the campaign in order for the staff to sell the advertised product. To me, this is a huge disconnect. Keep in mind, the people who develop the marketing campaign should have the advantage of knowing how to present that product or service to ensure the integrity of the brand. The company hired to launch the promotion must train the existing staff on how to present the promotional offer.

As an owner, you can never let a promotion company bring in an outside sales staff to present your health club. Building the relationship between the new member and the club is the key to building member loyalty. If an unknown salesperson sells the membership, and then your staff has to reengage the new member and try to build another relationship, it can make the new member feel as though he or she is being shuffled around. This reflects poorly on the club because the new member feels as though there is no stability or security within the business. It is even worse if the new member really connects with the salesperson and then discovers he or she is not going to be around in a month or so; the member will feel like a number as opposed to a valued member.

Throughout my years of traveling the country visiting clubs I have seen and heard the most outlandish sales presentations and representations of numerous clubs' memberships by outside sales staff. After the promotion company is gone, the owner and staff are left to clean up. I've had owners tell me the salespeople told prospects that the club was putting in a pool when the club was in a high-rise, or that the membership could be frozen or transferred, when the salesperson clearly knew the membership was nontransferable and could not be frozen. These fly-by-night hucksters will say anything to sell memberships and get their commissions because they know they will be down the road next month and couldn't care less about the carnage they leave behind.

As part of my program, I incorporate a professional-sales system that anyone can follow no matter his or her level of experience or skill set. In chapter three, I went through an in-depth sales system for locking up relationships, but it takes years to master that system, and each of my campaigns were only going to be forty-five to ninety days long at the very most. The duration of the campaign has to be short and sweet, otherwise you risk conditioning the market into thinking your membership is only worth X. This is another reason you can only incorporate a campaign like this into your marketing strategy if you are qualified to profile, engage, and lock up relationships with the deconditioned segment.

I don't have five years to teach a club's staff my entire system; besides, most people wouldn't learn it even if I laid it out step-by-step, as I have done in this book. The fact is, someone must love sales and marketing to give it the time it requires. I had to create a condensed version and incorporate the key points of the sale into my marketing materials so selling would now become order taking. Most clubs are plagued with staff issues, so my campaign's sales system had to be designed so any staff member in the club could take the order. The system had to be engineered so that there was no need for sales skills. I wanted to be able to assure my clients there would be no need for additional staff because anyone from a student at the front desk to the bookkeeper in the back office, could take the order with ease.

The only way I knew I could accomplish this was to ensure our marketing pieces and direct-mail pieces completely outlined the membership from cost to content. I knew there could be no miscommunication or confusion. I also wanted to involve the entire staff, from the front-counter person to the secretary in the back office, in the training, so they would know exactly what we were offering and how to take the order, so at no time was a prospect left waiting, and every staff member felt involved as an important part of the team. Involving the entire staff brings the team together for a common goal. I have always believed everyone in the club should be actively selling, or at least prospecting for the club. Employees must know their paychecks are dependent on the club's ability to bring in revenue, and it is everyone's responsibility to make sure the club is growing. At the same time, I believe everyone should be compensated for their effort, for example, a commission, bonuses, or perks.

If you spend time around me, you'll hear me say, "This is one of the reasons I have been successful," and if you are around me long enough, you'll hear me say it hundreds of times referencing hundreds of different things. With that preface, here I go again.

I feel one of the reasons I am so successful is I always put the other person first. I learned a long time ago that in any negotiation, if you unearth what the other person *really* wants first (I emphasize "really" because most people tell you one thing but mean another) and think of how you can give it to him or her, you should easily be able to find a way to get what you need as well. This is truly how it went with the design of MMC®'s compensation plan. I literally designed everything before I ever thought about how I was going to be paid. Had I done it the other way around—thinking of how much money I was going to charge first—I would have been putting the cart ahead of the horse. Look at it this way: How could I know the least I could accept until I knew exactly what it was going to cost me to produce and market the product?

Before you go into a negotiation, you must know what you can't live without and the very least you are willing to accept; everything else is negotiable. So I sharpened my pencil and started going through the figures.

Since I had already done my research and locked up pricing with all of the vendors, like the list company and the mailing house, I knew almost to a penny what my expenses would be. I was determined not to pass expenses on to my clients for things like market analyses, consumer profiling, and competitive overviews, because most owners would not have a frame of reference as to their importance relative to the success of the overall campaign and would therefore want to contest their necessity. There was no way I could get into this conversation every time I partnered with a new client to grow their business, because I knew two of the keys to the campaign's success were data and research. So, I had no choice but to factor these cost in to MMC®'s hard costs just as I did for personnel, office overhead, and so on.

I thought of the outrageous percentages the promotion companies collected in the past, which were basically as much as they could get but usually ended up between 40 and 60 percent above exaggerated expenses. Since there were no upgrades, add-ons, up sales, or back-end revenue increases, about 20 percent of the revenue was all the club owners received from the entire promotion. It seemed to me the scale was tipped too far in favor of the promotion company, which was only there for thirty days, whereas the owner had put his or her whole life into the club. I understand it was the promoter who came up with the idea, implemented it, and managed it, but it was the club owner who put his or her blood, sweat, and tears into the business. To me, those promotion-company owners were no better than common criminals who stole with a briefcase instead of a gun.

Just as I had to unearth the right price-point for the Cash campaign, I also had to determine a fair commission (or success fee) for MMC®. I was determined to find a number where the owner came out way on top, and I (the marketer) was treated fairly relative to my contribution and the value I brought to the business. Ironically, after running the numbers, the number I settled on was 20 percent of the total cash brought in from MMC®'s Cash campaign. We would receive no back-end revenue—revenue from profit centers or renewals—unless the club asked MMC® to run a renewal campaign. The club's annual back-end revenue would normally mirror the cash collected at the point of sale. For example, if the club raised $100,000 in cash, then the back-end revenue was projected to be $100,000 per year for the duration of the campaign. If the membership was for two years and the club brought in $100,000 in cash, the campaign is projected to generate another $100,000 each year, which meant the campaign would generate around an additional $200,000 in back-end revenue over the next two years, bringing the total revenue raised by MMC® to $300,000. But MMC® would be compensated only on the initial $100,000. In short, although MMC® was directly responsible for $300,000 in revenue, we are only paid on the $100,000 collected at the point of sale, making the real number being paid to MMC® more like 4 percent of the total revenue generated for the business. I felt this was a number no one could argue with.

Over the past twenty-five years, prices for everything have increased, but MMC® have never increased our commission. In 1991, it was 20 percent, and today in 2016, it is 20 percent. I am proud to say the same for MMC®'s vendors. Twenty-five years ago, we agreed on pricing, and although paper, wages, insurance policies, rents, and most all other business expenses have increased, our vendors have never raised their prices, because they were able to offset some costs thanks to new technology. The only prices that have increased for MMC®'s Cash campaign are those we have no control over: postage, local newspaper ads, radio advertisements, and so on. This is why building the right relationships with credible, competent people and companies are paramount to ensure the longevity of any business.

I was confident I would have no problem selling this "lost-leader" marketing concept of offering an introductory membership with a lower barrier-to-entry to an untapped segment of the market, because it was truly owner-friendly and absolutely the best marketing campaign the health-club industry had ever seen. It was nothing like those old promotions or companies; I had completely overhauled the model from top to bottom. I took all the risk out (risk reversal) by making the campaign completely self-funding and self-propelling. I eliminated any suspicion of fraud or misrepresentation, because no one in my company (including myself) ever collects one dime of the membership money being paid by the new member; the club's staff would collect all the money and deposit it into the owner's bank account, not ours. The club pays the vendors directly from the funds raised through the Cash campaign. The club pays MMC® its success fee every Monday from the previous week's revenue, so at no time would there be a question as to whether MMC® deserves payment or not; the proof is in the numbers. My Cash campaign includes tons of upgrades and add-ons for future growth ensuring the financial health of the business long-term. The campaign was absolutely a no-brainer—or was it?

CHAPTER 8

ON THE ROAD AGAIN

I had just spent the better part of five years constructing the greatest campaign that had ever been seen. Nowhere on earth could you find a legitimate, honest, legal, ethical way of making such a massive ROI than you could with my Cash campaign. Everyone won—the club owner won because he or she acquired new members with absolutely no risk and no money out of pocket, the campaign raises hundreds of thousands of dollars at the point of sale, and the traffic brings in a ton of revenue for the following two to three years. Member loyalty is guaranteed because these new members are in committed long-term relationships they love. Members win because they get to be part of a health club for a fraction of the published rates. The employees win because their clubs stays in business, providing them with long-term employment. I had no doubt in my mind once the word got out, every health club in America would be knocking on my door; all I was lacking was my first paying client.

Up until now, for a year or so, I had been running my campaigns for free for past clients and for the chain of clubs where I was employed as area director. Now that I had all of the bugs worked out, it was time for me to start looking for paying customers. I had invested almost every dime I had to my name on data, design, and testing the Cash campaign, and by this time, I was no longer working, so I needed to sell a club on this campaign quickly because I was becoming cash poor. Luckily, I had amassed an incredible line of unsecured credit, including credit cards with very high credit limits. I was never one for living above my means and rarely got upside down, but now, I was on the verge of having to get a job just to keep paying my bills. But I knew if I did, it could possibly derail or at a minimum, delay me from realizing my true calling. One of the reasons I was so successful is because I was really concerned with the good I could do for all Americans who wanted to join health clubs but couldn't afford it, as well as all those club owners who would lose everything they had worked their entire lives for if they didn't get some help fast. What I was doing would serve the greater good, so there was no way I could give up now. So once again, I packed my car with my clothes, my dog, and my guitar and headed down the road. (I know, my life sounds like a country song, but that's exactly the way it happened.)

By this time, I had spent most of my adult years traveling, so I wasn't worried in the least. I had also sold numerous clubs on the other promotion, and the Cash campaign I had engineered was far superior to anything an owner had ever seen before. I just needed to get on the road in a new city or state, because it would have been unethical to run a campaign for one of the competitors of the four clubs I had represented in Chicago, and the other clubs outside of their market were so conditioned to me running free campaigns for them, they weren't receptive to the idea of now paying me 20 percent of the gross—which I understood completely. It's only human nature to have pushback when the terms of the relationship change.

My strategy was to first visit all of the prospects I had met with in the past to show them how the promotion had evolved into the greatest marketing campaign unknown to the health-club industry and how my design and implementation were going to grow their businesses so fast their heads would spin. My Cash campaign was now a performance-based, data-driven, worry-free, turnkey member-acquisition campaign, specifically designed to acquire new members from an untapped segment through a no-risk self-funding marketing campaign. I had every objection in the world covered with rebuttals that would make my campaign a no-brainer—or so I thought.

As I drove from state to state, town to town, and club to club, I received one polite dismissal after another. One of the biggest hurdles was that the other companies claimed to put the money up to pay for the promotion, so clubs wondered why I wasn't fronting the money for my campaign. I explained that those old promotion companies only said they were fronting the money for the promotion but it was just a scam (smoke and mirrors), they only put up the money to send letters to present and past members, which costs a few hundred dollars, and then the money from their membership sales was what was funding the promotion. I also informed the club owners the promotion companies were exaggerating the expenses and the clubs were getting screwed by doing business the old way, but with my model, the owner would be in complete control. I showed the owners in detail how the old promoters were able to charge extravagant fees, like 50 percent and 60 percent above exaggerated expenses, just because they made it sound as if they were the ones who were paying for everything and taking all of the risk. It seemed the more I explained, the less the owners believed me. I even thought I sounded like a disgruntled ex-employee at times. Club owners were so blinded by the false narrative, "The promoter pays all of the expenses," they couldn't see it was all smoke and mirrors.

I told owners I could easily do the same and front the startup cost of my campaign (because even though I was running out of cash, I had a ton of credit cards), but it would be unethical and a lie when all I would be putting up would be a couple of hundred dollars to mail to expired members, and I refused to do it just to prove the club owner wrong.

Owners would often say, "If you are raising the revenue to fund the campaign by mailing to my past members, why can I not just do it on my own?" I would answer, "You can, if you want to be out of business next year, because you sold your memberships to health-conscious consumers at a price-point designed to bring in new business from an untapped market." My approach is to inform the current and past members of the offer but discourage them from migrating over while encouraging them to promote the introductory membership to their family and friends (birds of a father flock together). This simple truth cost me a fortune in lost commissions because of the naivety and greed of some owners.

Even today owners think they can run MMC®'s Cash campaign because they know a couple of details like price-point and the four phases of the campaign. There are hundreds if not thousands of details they don't know, but the most important of all is they don't know how to identify, engage and lock up relationships with the decondition segment, which is the most important component of this entire campaign. If you rollout a price-point like this without the pertinent information, you will only attract those customers who under normal circumstances would have easily paid the regular membership rate, but instead you will cannibalize your market and ruin your own business.

Another objection I often ran into was that the previous companies claimed to send in "professional" salespeople to the clubs to handle all of the sales so the clubs didn't have to rely on their untrained employees. I explained the old promotion companies only did that so they could collect the money coming through the door and deposit it into the promoters' bank accounts. I explained how most of those "professional" salespeople were just local hires (with one or two from the home office) with absolutely no experience in sales, or even in the club business, for that matter. I always stressed that I had removed the need for a sales staff altogether and that my Cash campaign require order-taking skills and not sales skills, but I was also going to train the club's staff for future growth just the same. But they were still set on me sending a sales staff in to sell all memberships. I could have easily hired a couple of people for $400 a week just to take the orders, but this would be terrible for the clubs, and even though I was going broke trying to educate these owners and could have closed some deals immediately had I just conceded, I couldn't bring myself to go against what was best for their businesses.

This went on for several months, and by then, my credit cards were maxed out, and I felt as if my butt was being handed to me. I couldn't figure it out to save my life. I started recording my presentations to see where I was dropping the ball. Was I saying something wrong? Was I not saying something? Was I speaking too fast? Was I speaking too slowly? Was I not listening? Was I talking too much? I was dumbfounded. Then, I started questioning the campaign. Should I claim to put up the money? Should I hire a local college kid to take the orders? Should I collect the money, put it in my bank account, and then send the owner his or her percentage after I kept the lion's share? Should I charge 40 or 50 percent? Did 20 percent make CTC look less professional because I was willing to take far less money than other companies? I started questioning the way I was dressed, the way I walked, and the way I combed my hair. I basically questioned every aspect of my existence. Fortunately, every time I started to doubt myself, I would recall a time in my life when I was facing insurmountable odds, and because I refused to give up or give in, I always rose to the occasion, so I stuck to my convictions and pressed on.

One night, I was in my hotel room, thinking of prospects I could call on, and a guy who owned a really nice athletic club in South Carolina came to mind. I had met with this guy back when I worked for the new promoter, and the club owner and I had hit it off well, but he just wasn't sold on the fire-sale promotion. He had literally built his club with his own two hands, and it was a family business as well as a second home to some terrific employees. He treated everyone like family, and all of his members and employees loved him. I remembered one of his objections had been that he didn't want to alienate his staff or take commissions out of his salesperson's pocket. In short, he didn't want outside salespeople coming into his club and taking over. He really understood the dynamics between his staff and the members, and he wasn't about to disrupt the chemistry of the club. He also wasn't sold on the price-point, and he had a few other concerns as well. This owner and I were on the same page when it came to customer service, so I thought about calling him, but it would be easy for him to blow me off over the phone. I knew if I could get in front of him, face to face, we could do something together, so early the next morning, I headed south.

When I arrived at his club, his front-counter person told me he was down the street at a local park, playing kickball with some employees and friends. So, I jumped in my car and drove to the park. When I got there, I looked like a duck out of water. I was wearing an Italian suit in South Carolina in the middle of summer, with what seemed like 100 percent humidity, but by that point, I didn't care what I looked like; I just needed work. So, I took off my jacket, loosened up my tie, rolled up my sleeves, walked over, and sat on the bleachers, sweating my butt off to watch the game. Of course, I was wearing a suit to make my best impression, but in hindsight, I looked like a doofus in that park that day. But I know now the owner liked that I was willing to be a team player, even if I was overdressed.

After the game was over, I went up, said hello, and asked the club owner whether I could take him to lunch so we could talk, and he accepted. Over lunch, he shared with me his concerns (which were pretty much the same as I remembered) about the promotion I had presented some time before and told me he had given it a lot of thought but had decided to go in a different direction with his marketing. He was a bit taken aback when I exclaimed, "Fantastic!" I went on to inform him why it had been so long since he had heard from me and then shared the changes I had made in my career as well as those I had made to the old fire-sale promotion. I went through all of the differences, and he became re-engaged in the conversation. I asked him how business was at the moment (a rhetorical question because I already knew the answer, since it was the middle of the summer), and he said business was slow. We left lunch that day agreeing to meet the following day at the club for a formal sit-down and presentation.

The following day, I entered the club and was directed upstairs to his office. After some pleasantries, we got right down to business. His concerns were the same as when I had met him before, and I was able to reiterate what I had explained to him at lunch the previous day, but today, he was a lot more receptive to my ideas much more than he had been previously. People love consistency; it is ingrained in our DNA through evolution. It's called the consistency principle. Consistency releases dopamine, which is the pleasure chemical in our brains, and inconsistency, suppresses dopamine. Inconsistency makes us very uncomfortable. That is why you must always be consistent with your customers throughout the entire relationship. It is so deeply rooted in our brains it will always be a game changer. People believe a familiar statement. This is why you must be consistent in your presentations. For people to become familiar with a statement, you must repeat it at least three times. Don't say it exactly the same way each time, but convey your point three different ways while saying the same thing. We need consistency in our lives. When we get pleasure, we want to experience it again and again. It is the familiarity with the message, person, place, thing, smell, and so on that takes over and makes us feel good.

Since I was able to gather pertinent information during the lunch the day before, I knew what my hurdles were and had used the rest of the day and night to design a presentation that guaranteed a win-win. Of course, the first question I asked myself was, how can I give him what he wants without diminishing the value of my campaign and without compromising my beliefs? Having the ability to compromise is an essential component of success. If you are going to be successful, you must know when and how to compromise and be flexible. The only time I refuse to compromise is when it comes to my morals and values. In this scenario, I was willing to compromise as long as it did not compromise the integrity of the Cash campaign.

When you first start your business, you need to get customers to use your product and testify to its success. Getting your first client is always the hardest, so be prepared to be flexible, especially in the beginning. After you have a proven track record, it is much easier to stand your ground.

I was able to address and provide a win-win solution to every one of his concerns without affecting the integrity of the campaign, just by presenting the same components of the campaign in different ways and in different lights. The only thing I changed was I would stay in South Carolina and not only implement and manage the campaign but I would also sell memberships along with his staff. I have discovered in life everything always turns out for the best, and this decision was one of those times. My pushback to having an outside salesperson in the club was that it didn't allow the staff to initiate and cultivate relationships with new members. This is far more important than you may think. Member loyalty is a buzzword now, but it has always been a primary concern for owners. Consistency is a powerful tool in building relationships, and you must do your best to keep your key personnel so when new members come to the club, they see familiar faces. So, to maintain consistency, I made it a point to let the new members know I too was a guest in the club and was just helping out with the campaign for a couple of months, and after I finished the paperwork,

I always introduced the new member to the club's key players, just to ensure the member got to know the club's staff. Although it would have been better not to have an outside salesperson at all, I was professional enough to pull it off because by then, I was familiar with the dynamics of the club.

Part of the agreement was the club would provide my lodging through a trade with a local hotel. I am pleased to say this club owner was a stand-up guy. He put me in a Marriott Residence Inn in a great part of town. By this point, most of my credit cards had been maxed out, as well as my lines of unsecured credit, so I was elated since the room came with some great perks, like meals. If you are not familiar with this hotel chain, it specializes in upscale apartment living. The place was huge, and since I had my dog (Seabreez, a Great Pyrenees) with me in my car, I welcomed the extra space; it had all the comforts of home. I knew I had made a great decision to compromise and stay in South Carolina, and I felt extremely lucky to have signed my first contract with such a fabulous club, a great owner, and a terrific staff. I respect the owner so much I named my third son after him more than fifteen years after the campaign, and I am still grateful to him for giving me a chance, even to this day.

I started the campaign immediately, and it took off like a rocket. The owner was a champ and let me run it exactly the way I designed it, and it rocked. The club brought in $250,000 in cash, and the club was rockin' in the middle of summer. Everyone loved the campaign, especially the members. Some of my fondest memories of being in the club business are of the people and friendships I built in that club. Yes, the campaign was a grand slam, and it was my first huge success (I had raised over $200,000 in a month for numerous clubs in the past, but this was the first time I had ever brought in $250,000 in cash at the point of sale), which proved I was correct about my theories. I was extremely happy I stuck to my guns when it came to the implementation of the campaign. As I am writing this book, I realize it was the education I took with me that was far more memorable and valuable than the monetary rewards. Two of my greatest lessons in my life come to mind.

One day, the club owner and I were talking, and he said, "Chuck, you are from Chicago. Why don't you dress nicer?" I was a little taken aback because I thought I was dressed appropriately. This was around 1990, and warm-up suits were really popular on the streets of Chicago—especially Michael Jordan's line of warm-up suits from Nike—and I had every one that Nike put out. When I was presenting a club, I wore a white shirt, suit and tie, but day to day, I wore Jordan head to toe. So, to say the least, the club owner's statement perplexed me, but I admired him and respected his observation, so I gave it serious thought. Then, it dawned on me: all the club staff, including the owner, were preppy dressers. They all wore khaki shorts or slacks with golf shirts. So, the next day, I went to the mall and changed my entire day-to-day wardrobe. I wasn't changing my style for them; I was changing my style for me and my future. If I was going to be in this business, I needed to dress as if I belonged to one of the tribe. Dress to impress, but also dress to mirror your prospects.

Another valuable lesson I took with me was love for the game of golf. Up until that point in my life, I hated the idea of golfing. I've always loved and studied full-contact sports, like football, martial arts, and boxing. The idea of hitting a little ball around a field sounded painful to me. If picking up your opponent and body-slamming him onto a bunker every time he duffed a ball had been in the rules, I would have been all in, but short of that, you could have the game. But I met a guy who worked at the club in Columbia who had just graduated from college, and he loved golf.

This guy's future was set. He looked exactly like Tom Cruise and had one of the hottest tiny southern belles in South Carolina as his fiancée. This girl was smokin' hot and super sweet, she came from an upscale family who owned one of the top-ten new golf courses in the South at the time, and he loved golf more than anything else, including women, which was a sin in my eyes. Every year, he organized a charitable golf outing that had a couple of hundred golfers' participation. He was a real stand-up guy who loved the game and wanted to share his passion with everyone.

Anyway, he and I got along great because he was extremely ambitious and wanted to learn sales and marketing. Every day, he would ask me to play golf with him, and I just wasn't interested in wasting four hours of my day on golf. I had a negative association with the game because of my history with club owners who preferred to be on the golf course instead of in their clubs, growing their businesses. But this guy was relentless, and one day, I gave in and said I would play a round with him.

I asked him what the best course in town to play was, and he told me but with a disclaimer that we could never play it because it was closed to the public and only open to members—ultraexclusive. I told him to be ready to golf and that we would play our first round at that country club the following week. He laughed his butt off, and then I saw the light come on, and he realized I was serious.

Since I am very competitive and think of myself as an athlete, I was not about to play a round without at least knowing the basics, so that evening, I set up a few lessons. Within a couple of lessons, I could hit the ball fairly well and was ready for my first round. I also called the country club and told them a friend and I were interested in visiting the club to inquire about membership (to be clear, I never said I was interested in joining), and as I knew they would, they set me up with an early-morning tee time as well as a complimentary breakfast for two. I don't remember the exact day, but I do know it was early in the week, like a Tuesday or a Wednesday, because after a little research, I knew the course would be easier to get on because most golfers want to golf on the weekends.

For those of you who want to know how to get the biggest discounts on memberships, always join in the slowest times of the year. Health clubs, as well as all other membership-based businesses, put out their best deals during their slow seasons. Never join a health club in January, because you'll pay a premium. Most clubs base their entire yearly budgets on January, February, and March sales. Inquire in June, July, or August, when clubs are dead. If you want to work out in a club and avoid the guest fee, go on a Friday, Saturday, or Sunday. These are the slowest days and usually have the weakest staff, which rarely check membership cards or follow procedures. If you do get someone who is on the ball, smile and ask about membership. You may have to sit through a presentation, but odds are you'll get a free workout.

It was picturesque that early morning on the first tee box. Light dew glimmered on the greens and fairways. At that very moment, I fell in love with the game of golf. I could now understand his passion for it. It was so much more than a sport; it was a lifestyle. We laughed and joked the entire time (mostly about how poorly I played). We literally had the course to ourselves, and it was one of the greatest memories of my life watching him explode with joy that morning at being able to share his love of the game with me. We finished our round and then had breakfast in the club's restaurant; this Tom Cruise look-alike was in complete disbelief the entire time. I explained to him golf courses have to raise revenue just like any other business, and since it is a member-based model, they too are always looking for new members. Even if a club has a waiting list, it will often entertain prospective members to get them on the list. I also got lucky because there are not a lot of golfers wanting to play golf in the middle of the summer in the South Carolina heat.

This guy with the movie-star looks taught me a ton about golf, and I could tell you so many funny stories about our golfing adventures, but I'll end with one more story. In those years, I loved to drink beer and party at night, and although he wasn't a big drinker, he came out with me every night. This, of course, did not sit well with his fiancée. One morning after an all-night of drinking, he came into the club looking as if he had just watched his dog get shot right in front of him. I asked him what on earth was wrong, and he said that when he had gotten home last night, he had seen a note from his fiancée that read, "Just marry Chuck since you prefer to spend all of your time with him"; she was breaking off the engagement. I was floored. On the one hand, it was funny as hell, because I had told him a girl like that would never put up with our crap, and he better start going home, but on the other hand, I felt really bad for him because I knew he loved her. I believe everything happens for the best, and a few years later, he met and married a wonderful girl.

One day, the receptionist at the club informed me I had a call from the owner of a club across town. The man introduced himself and informed me he owned a couple of clubs. One of his clubs was built for a condominium complex and was way off the beaten path, and because of its poor location, it was struggling. He wanted to know whether I thought my Cash campaign could work there. I informed him I couldn't discuss the campaign with him, because of my loyalty to the club owner of this first club where I was currently running my Cash campaign, and he said he respected that but the first owner was the one who had given him my name. I took his information and told him after I spoke with the first owner and did a little research on the second owner's club I would get back to him. So I spoke to the first club owner, and he asked me to help the second club owner, he stated they weren't direct competitors, and said they had been friends for years. After some research, I informed the second owner the Cash campaign would work, but because of some of the information I got back from the data, it was likely to only bring in about $150,000. The second owner said that would be fantastic, so we set up the Cash campaign to be launched one week after the first club's closeout.

This condominium club was an old racquetball-court club set way in the back of all the other businesses and commercial buildings which were just off a main road. It was really out of the way, and prospects had to make an effort to go back there, but I had the secret sauce to get them to do just that. Immediately, I got to work training the staff on how to professionally sell a membership. We still had about two weeks before the direct mail would hit, and we were struggling to get past members to rejoin. I convinced the owner to tear out a couple of racquetball courts so we could add more equipment and enlarge the aerobic area. This minor investment paid off huge dividends. The renewals picked up, and the place started to rock once the direct mail hit.

One day, I was driving up to the club's entrance as the owner was leaving. He invited me to grab a bite so we could discuss the business. As we sat down, he started the conversation off by thanking me for the success of the campaign and asked what he could do to keep growing the club after I was gone. I shared some things with him about additional marketing and customer service. He was really fortunate because his son and daughter worked at the club, and even though they had been raised with money, they were both very cool, down-to-earth and the members loved them. So, I had to address the business side of customer service only in reference to member retention, and not staffing issues. On our ride home, I commented on his car because it was a beautiful Mercedes Benz; he said thanks and kind of chuckled. I asked him why he chuckled (we had built a friendship during the month I had been in his club), and he said he was just thinking about my Cadillac. I said, "What about my Caddy?" At this time in my life I owned a black Cadillac Coupe Deville.

He said, "Do you know what people think when they see a guy pull up in a Cadillac?"

I answered no. He said a Cadillac tells people you are a redneck who made a little bit of money. He continued by saying a man who grew up with wealth doesn't wear it around his neck or on his fingers. I knew he was referring to guys who wore diamond rings and gold chains around their necks, which is typical of guys who own Cadillacs. He was right, and I knew it. When I lived in Chicago, I wore a diamond-cut gold Saint Christopher necklace (the patron saint of travel). I didn't wear rings, but I got the message loud and clear. The night I lost that necklace, I was in a sports bar on the northwest side of Chicago. I had gotten into a bar fight with some guys over a pool game. The next day, I had woken up to my girlfriend screaming her head off because I was covered in blood. It looked a lot worse than it was because I had passed out in a solid-white Jordan warm-up suit. When I got my clothes off, I saw I had been stabbed in the side of my calf, and it had bled badly, but other than that, I was fine. The necklace had been ripped off my neck in the fight, and I never replaced it because I wasn't that guy anymore.

A few weeks later, the second club's closeout was done, raising around $180,000 in cash, and the owner couldn't have been happier. After South Carolina, I worked with a club in Georgia and then somehow, I got a lead down in Jacksonville, Florida, so I was headed even further south. This was going to be my fourth club and it was time to remove myself from the club's daily operations.

I set this Cash campaign up where I would stay in Jacksonville near the club, but I would only be the project manager. I would train the staff, as I had originally designed the campaign, and the existing staff would be the ones to take all of the orders (do the sales). The owner was cool with this because he knew of the enormous success I had in the three previous clubs and was just elated to have me there; later, I discovered the reason why he was so elated.

This campaign too went off as planned, and soon, the racquet club was a real health club, filled with excitement and new members. Things were going great in my business life, but every time I opened the door of my Caddy, those words of "rich redneck" rang in my ears. I couldn't take it any longer, and one day, I drove straight to a BMW dealership and bought a 700 series. Presentation is everything, and although I am a firm believer in American-made products, I was not going to be prejudged before I ever got out of my car. Most people in the health-club business came from the same backgrounds, wore the same clothes, drove the same cars, and to most of their demises, ran their businesses the same way. I would never be able to accomplish my goals if I was presenting myself as someone completely unlike them—an outsider wearing warm-up suits with tacky jewelry and driving a pimpmobile. So, I retired the Caddy for good. From that day forward, I wore a blue blazer with starched white shirts and Robert Talbott ties for presentations, cargo shorts or khaki pants and polo shirts or button-downs for every day, and the only jewelry I wore was a Rolex watch. The funny thing was, it felt completely natural.

I fell in love with Jacksonville. The club owner owned a chain of martial arts schools and loved golf, so we hit it off fast. One day, he came to my office and asked me to play a round with him, and of course, I said yes. He then told me not to tell anyone in the club, which I thought was a bit odd. Later, on the course, I asked him why he hadn't wanted anyone to know we were golfing, and he said even though he owned the club, when people saw him leave to go play golf, they felt slighted because they had to stay and work. That was news to me because I loved to work, and I never would have thought employees could feel that way. When I was in the clubs and the owner went to golf, I just thought he didn't have his priorities straight, but never did I envy him but it was good to get a different perspective on employees.

I played golf because I really loved the game, and now, it was becoming a business tool, but it was still very difficult for me to take five hours out of my day (drive time plus a four-hour round). Within just a couple of years of learning, I went to playing only nine holes, and then even, nine holes became rare just because of the time the game consumed. I love working, and a golf course is not the appropriate place for taking calls and working out ideas. Most golfers I know golf for relaxation or to socialize, and I relax best after a hard day's work and am not a big fan of socializing outside of my family, so nowadays, I may play nine holes with my kids every now and then, but that's about as much golf as I get in.

There was a Mexican restaurant near the athletic club, and I started dating this little Mexican lady who loved Jacksonville. She took me everywhere and showed me all of the sites, and I fell in love with the city. Officially, I was living in Los Angeles at the bottom of the Hollywood Hills, which is where I had rented an apartment to have an address, but I hadn't been there in months, because my home was the road. I chose Los Angeles for the presentation of my brand. Everyone thinks of California as being the leader in fitness. Back then, the East Coast was actually much further ahead of the West Coast when it came to the business of health clubs. But perception is people's reality, and if they perceived Los Angeles as being the hot spot for fitness and health-club experts, then I wanted to have a Los Angeles address.

The Jacksonville club did very well, but there were a few hiccups along the way. After the first week, I went to cash my commission check, and the bank told me the club's account had been frozen by the IRS. I went to the owner and asked him what was up, and he told me he was working everything out and to please give him one week to fix it. A week later, I got my money, and since the campaign brought in a lot of cash, it got the guy out of his financial jam. I really enjoyed working with that club and the owner; as always, I learned a lot, but it was time to go once again. After the Jacksonville club's closeout, I went on the road selling campaigns.

Now that I had four solid testimonials, it was easier to get club owners to listen and give my Cash campaign a shot. I did several promotions and rarely made it back to Los Angeles because most of my clients were on the East Coast. I decided to move to Jacksonville and hire the Mexican girl as my secretary. By this time, the relationship was strictly a friendship, and I needed someone I could trust to handle my banking and all other aspects of my financial affairs. She had a college degree and was super smart as well as loyal, and those were the two most important characteristics to me.

As I stated earlier, I am a lover of learning, and I believe people's futures are impacted by two things: nature and nurture. Humans are born with certain characteristics (nature), and we develop certain characteristics through nurture. Steadfast, independent, honest, sensible, down-to-earth, imaginative, creative, hardworking, practical, business-minded, enthusiastic, analytical, loyal, and truthful are all adjectives that have been used to describe me and are characteristics I nurture daily. I know I was born to serve others and to do it honestly. This was the reason I liked this little chili pepper in Jacksonville—her honesty.

She was loyal and a very good person. She should have worked for Jacksonville's tourism department because she was the one who sold me on moving to Jacksonville. I rented a townhouse and started operating my business from two of the bedrooms I had turned into offices. After settling in, I was back on the road selling campaigns. Today, life is so much easier because of YouTube and the Internet. Back in the 1990s, if you didn't knock on doors and have face-to-face meetings, you didn't close deals. It wears a person down being on the road. I always had two sets of luggage: one with me, and one with clean clothes waiting at home by the door. Sometimes, I would literally walk through the front door, drop my bags, pick up the other set, turn around, and go right back out again. This was my lifestyle for about fifteen years.

Just as I had in the past for the promotion companies, I drove from coast to coast, north to south, crisscrossing the entire lower forty-eight states, rarely leaving the road during the first decade of MMC®. There was no budget for rental cars, flights, or five-star hotels. I was grinding it out in the trenches, melting the rubber off my tires, eating cheap greasy fast food, sleeping in motels (not hotels), and living from promo to promo. I would spend entire days in my motel room making cold calls to clubs when I didn't have an appointment. There weren't any cell phones that I could afford to use for that many calls and minutes every day. I had a cell phone, but the cost per minute was absurd; my cell was only for emergency calls. I would meet a lady somewhere on the road, and she would say, "Gosh, it must be so great traveling everywhere, seeing all these new places, and meeting so many new people," and I would think to myself, Huh, if you only knew. I wasn't taking family trips to Disneyland; I was driving to work. People complain about having to commute to work for thirty minutes in traffic; my daily commute was hours and hundreds of miles every day.

One summer, I was going on a road trip through the South and stopped in Jacksonville to pick up fresh clothes, and my secretary asked me whether she and her daughter could tag along for a week since her daughter was out of school for summer vacation. I knew this was a bad idea; they thought it was going to be fun and games when in reality, it was extremely difficult, but I still said yes. We (I) drove all over North Carolina, South Carolina, and Georgia and had one last appointment in Lake Charles, Louisiana. We were just outside of Atlanta, and if we drove all night, I'd make my early-morning appointment on time. Around four in the morning, I was exhausted and asked my secretary whether she felt she could drive us on into Lake Charles without falling asleep so I could lie in the back and take a nap. She said absolutely. I told her daughter to make sure she kept talking to her mom so she wouldn't fall asleep behind the wheel, and she said no problem. I climbed in the back seat and closed my eyes.

No sooner I was in a deep sleep than I felt us spinning as though we were on a teacup ride at the county fair. I heard screeching tires and blowing horns. I rose up, and my secretary was asleep behind the wheel. I started screaming her name to wake her up as we crossed the westbound lanes on I-10, narrowly missing other cars. When we hit the median, she woke and tried to straighten the car but overcorrected and shot us back across the westbound lanes. We ended up crashing in a ditch on the far side of the westbound lanes. I asked the girls whether they were OK, and they both were. Luckily, none of us had a scratch, and since it was just before dawn, there were few cars on the interstate. I got out and checked the car, and it was totaled. The tires were bent underneath the car, and it wasn't going anywhere.

A car stopped, and the driver asked us whether we were all right, and we said we were. Now that we were all fine, my mind was back on business and my appointment. I asked the driver whether he would give us a ride to the next exit with a hotel, and he said of course. I told the girls to grab what they could carry, and we took off. Up ahead just a couple of miles was an exit with a hotel. We checked in, and I told my secretary to call a tow truck and a taxi. I jumped in the shower and took a taxi to the club. I arrived on time and closed the deal. I then took a taxi back to the hotel, got the girls, went to the airport, and rented a van to drive back to Jacksonville. That was years ago. I still have the same secretary, and not once has she or her daughter ever asked to go on the road with me again.

Speaking of crazy road trips, one time, I had an appointment with a club in New Jersey, and I was running low on funds. I had barely enough money for my airfare and hotel. My flight was to Newark Airport, and I was going to jump on a bus to get to the hotel and then take a taxi to the club the following morning. I couldn't drive my car up to Jersey, because if I had the slightest mechanical problem, I would have been stranded because I wouldn't have had the money to fix it. This was also during the time I was trying to rebuild my credit, so I didn't have a credit card with enough credit to rent a car. As my flight neared Newark Airport, the captain came over the loudspeaker and announced there was a problem and we were being diverted to Philly. I couldn't believe it. I barely had enough money for a snack, and now I had to figure out how in the world I was going to make it from Philly to Jersey. I knew the airline would give me a ticket from Philly to Jersey, book me on another flight, cover my hotel bill, and give me a food voucher (those were the good ole days when airlines knew what customer service was), but that would cause me to leave Philly the following day, and I couldn't take the chance of missing the appointment, because I really needed the sale. Frantically, I start asking the other passengers whether anyone was driving up to Jersey. One of the passengers said I could catch a ride with him to the train station; there, I could get a train. Great, there went my hotel money as well as a good night's sleep. Canceled flights, lost car-rental reservations, fully booked hotels, and on and on just knocks the wind out of you, but if you want to be a successful salesperson, it is part of the job.

When I first started CTC (Chuck Thompson Consulting) before MMC®, I required a $2,500 retainer (which would be deducted from the first commissions) when signing with a club. After a couple of years, I stopped that practice so there would be absolutely no up-front fees associated with my Cash campaign. In the initial setup, I would be underwater for the first couple of weeks, so I needed a security deposit (retainer) to guarantee the club wouldn't bail on me before I at least recuperated a portion of my initial investment for their consumer profile.

I was flying up to Jersey with just enough money to make it to the appointment with the club owner, and if I didn't close this deal, I would be walking back to the airport, but at least I had a return ticket to Jacksonville. When I got to the train station in Philadelphia, I was told the next train didn't leave until morning, but if I got a hotel room, I wouldn't have had the money for the train ticket. So, I sat down, got my book from my bag, and started reading until I got tired enough to get some shut-eye while I waited for the next train.

My appointment was early in the morning, and by the time the train got me to Jersey, the time was getting really tight. The club was a good distance from the station, so I jumped in a cab and told the driver where I was going. As we were driving, I kept my eyes on the meter, and when we got close to the end of my money, I told the driver to stop, and I got out. I was still a couple of miles from the club, so I started running. In my entire career, I had never been late for a meeting or missed a meeting, and I wasn't about to start. I was in fabulous shape, so it was no big deal for me to run a couple of miles, but I was getting really hungry, and I didn't want to take the chance of spending any of the money I had left, in case I needed it later. In no time, I was near the club, so I stopped and went in a restaurant to freshen up in the bathroom. I had brought my suit in a garment bag, so I hung it on the stall door, washed in the sink, and changed clothes in the stall. I brushed my teeth, combed my hair and went to the club looking as though I had spent the night in the downtown Marriott.

The club was on a major thoroughfare, which is always good news, and the club's layout was well designed; you could see the fit, sexy members from the road through the plate-glass windows. Of course, the club was empty because it was around nine in the morning. The owner's son met me and showed me around the club. This guy was really nice, and I could see he not only loved to work out but also loved the health-club business. His dad was an elderly gentleman and very serious, the kind of guy who is strictly business and no BS. His son, on the other hand, was making jokes and flirting with the girls on staff and the few female members who were in the club, and I could see the father was getting annoyed with his son because he wanted to get down to business. It was funny; I used to be just like the son, but now that I owned my own business and had all the responsibilities on my shoulders, I saw myself in the dad. We got into the meat and potatoes of the campaign, and they both loved the idea. Within a couple of hours, I was walking to their bank and cashing my retainer check. That Jersey club brought in $177,000 in immediate cash within just thirty days.

Thinking about that Jersey club reminds me of another Jersey club. I was on the road in northern New Jersey, just across the Ben Franklin Bridge from Philly, and I had an appointment with an owner of a well-known gym. Whenever possible, if I was traveling somewhere, I always tried to set up appointments with every club in the area so I saw all the competition, drove around the area, got a feel for the demographics, which also increased my odds of closing a deal that day. So, as I was turning off the main road to go back to see this gym owner, I saw a beautiful athletic club just off the main road. Without ever seeing the inside, I knew straight away that athletic club would crush the gym in numbers if I ran a campaign for it, simply because of the location. I had an hour or so before my appointment with the gym, so I decided to drop in and see whether the owner was available. Remember the three rules of real estate: location, location, and location.

The club was huge and packed with the latest equipment. It was an old tennis club, and the owner had taken several courts out and converted the space into a fitness floor. It was done very well, and the place was hopping in the middle of the day with what we refer to today as soccer moms. The owner was the stereotypical Jersey guy, with a muscle T-shirt, gold jewelry, and a foul mouth. We sat down, and not five minutes into the presentation, he started shouting, "I'd never do this f——in' program. You're ruining the f——in' industry. Get the f—— out of my club." I was so tempted to knock this loudmouth out, but I had become a different person, and I was there representing MMC®. The image of my company was far more important to me now than my macho ego. So, I smiled, gathered my things, thanked him for his time, and left the building. I left thinking to myself, he doesn't know how lucky he is to still have teeth, but it wasn't over yet. I had a much harder punch for his loud mouth. I went to the gym, which was less than a mile away, for my next appointment. I was going to do their campaign (even if I had to do it for free) and bankrupt that loudmouth down the street.

The gym owner was waiting for me at the counter with a huge smile. He was really short and huge from steroids, but this young guy knew what he wanted out of life and was willing to work his butt off to get it. He was a businessman first and a gym rat second. He had a great club with a similar history to the athletic club up the street, only this was an old racquetball club that had been converted into a cool gym. I was thinking, when I launch this campaign, it is going to bring down the pain on that loudmouth at the athletic club. The club owner and I spent about an hour together, addressing his concerns and laying out the campaign, and then, we went straight into the paperwork. I launched that gym's campaign immediately, and it sold over a thousand memberships and brought in more than $200,000 in immediate cash. Normally, every Monday, I am happy to see the sales reports so I can pay some bills, but during this campaign, I just wanted to see how many members I was keeping from joining the athletic club up the street. I am a firm believer that when you seek revenge, you should dig two graves: one for your enemy, and one for yourself. But this was different; this club owner was completely out of hand. A few years earlier, he would have been eating through a straw for six weeks, but this was business; I was doing the best job I could for my client, and the little payback I was getting was just a by-product of a job well done.

About a year later, my secretary told me a club owner wanted to speak to me about the campaign. She gave me the name, and wouldn't you know it, it was that Jersey athletic club owner. I picked up the phone and instantly said, "Is this so-and-so? I thought you would never f——in' do my campaign. I thought I was ruining the f——in' industry. Why are you calling me?"

He said, "Chuck, I'm really sorry I was a prick that day, but man, your campaign killed me, and I lost a lot of my members to the gym, and I really need your help." Wow, I didn't expect him to humble himself like that, and now my thoughts went from anger to immediate empathy. I told him I was really sorry, but his club was just too close to the gym, and I couldn't run a campaign for one of my client's competitors; I felt bad for the guy and actually gained a little respect for him because he had the cojones to admit he was wrong. A few months later, the gym owner sold his club. This athletic club owner called me back, and MMC® ended up running the Cash campaign for him. It didn't do anywhere near as well as the gym had, because at that point I hadn't developed other options for the Cash campaign like MMC® has today, so it was exactly the same campaign targeting the same demographic with the same price-point. I think we ended up just over $100,000, but it was still good enough for him because he got back most of his members plus some new ones.

MMC® was growing, I had finally gotten my finances and credit back in shape, and life was good. I was doing a ton of business by now, most of it coming from referrals, although I pounded the market with advertising, especially direct mail, to keep our name in owners' minds. I had worked out all the kinks, and it was very rare for a promotion not to hit the numbers I projected. But on occasion, something would arise and really make me scratch my head, like a promotion I was running for a club in Torrance, California. This club was in a terrific area, the owner was hands on, and the club had all of the amenities. The owner was in good shape financially but was always looking for ways to bring in new business and had heard about MMC® from another club we had worked with, so he wanted to give us a shot. He and I hit it off right away. He loved golf and drove a big Caddy. I had been driving a Mercedes

Benz for a while by this time, but I still loved and missed the roominess of a Caddy. I knew this club was a home run and would easily bring in a quarter of a million dollars in no time at all.

I launched the first phase of the campaign, and it caught on like wildfire. As I was running the first phase, my team (by now I could afford a team) was preparing for the direct mail phase of the campaign. Normally, we can judge when mail is going to hit people's mailboxes and when the subsequent rush of people is going to flood the club. That day came, and we were ready, but nothing happened. I told the staff not to worry, because the post office has about ten business days to get the mail out, so the mail should hit mailboxes any day. The next day came, and there was not one phone call. The next day, not one phone call either. Then the fourth, the fifth—this went on for about two weeks. By this time, my new golfing buddy wasn't so pleasant and wanted to know where his mail was; I didn't show it, but I was wondering the same thing. I got on the phone and started calling our people, our vendors, the post offices, and anyone else I thought I could get some answers from. Luckily, my mailing house has great relationships with postmasters all over the United States and our representative was able to get ahold of the postmaster for Torrance and was informed the mail truck carrying our mail had been in an accident and had been impounded.

My team went to work on resolving the issue and got the mail out, and boom, the club exploded. We did over $300,000 for that business, and the owner loved us. In fact one day, I was in the club in the owner's office, and a call came in for me, which kind of shocked me because my office would have called my cell. It was a lady who owned a women-only club up the hill, wanting me to run a campaign for her. The owner I was currently working with had given her my name and had his secretary let her know when I was in his office. He gave me the green light, and I brought in over $150,000 for her little women's-only club not two miles from his athletic club. I remember him saying, "Help her out if you can, Chuck, because she and I are not competitors. We have completely different products and markets." Of course, I disagreed and voiced my opinion, but he was super nice and really wanted me to help her, so I did.

California is a great state, and I do a ton of business there. One day, I got a call from a club in West Hollywood wanting MMC® to run a campaign for them. Normally, I try to close the sale over the phone, especially if the club has been referred to me, but this guy really wanted me to come out and see him, so I caught a flight out and went to his club. Previously, I had lived at the foot of the Hollywood Hills; West Hollywood was really nice, but that was about all I knew of the area and since I had lived not far from this club years ago—I didn't see reason to do any preliminary research because I knew any club in that area would do well. I walked into the club, and it was packed with really good-looking guys. The owner greeted me and introduced himself, all the while looking me up and down. He said, "Let me show you around," and as we toured the club, I noticed there wasn't one woman in the entire place. As we entered the locker room, I saw a bunch of enlarged photographs on the wall of buff men who happened to be completely naked. It is very normal to see pictures, posters, and paintings of buff guys as motivation and inspiration in most clubs, but I had never seen pictures of naked men, and then, bam! We turned the corner, and out on the sundeck were a half-dozen naked men sunbathing. I noticed the owner watching me to see whether I was about to lose it, but I kept my cool, and we continued the tour. When we sat down in his office, he said, "You obviously know by now we are a health club that serves the gay community. Have you ever promoted a gay club before?" I said no, I hadn't—yet. He said he knew all about MMC® and our campaign, and the only thing he needed to know from me was whether I thought I could make it work there and target just men. I said, "Absolutely."

Club owners don't understand what profiling is when it comes to consumers. My team can profile any demographic by their spending habits and buying patterns, just as novices use rudimentary demographic data by looking for age, gender, income, and education, you can create an algorithm to produce an avatar of your ideal customer and build your profile around that avatar's spending habits and lifestyle choices. Today, Google, Amazon, and other online companies start building customer profiles of all of their customers from the very first time the consumer makes a purchase from their sites. Back in the 1980s and 1990s, the data cost a fortune, but my team and I were the pioneers in profiling consumers for health-club memberships. Today, it is a lot cheaper and easier if you have the profile, know what to look for, where to get the data, and how to interpret the data. But even in the 1990s, the data was available; you just had to know what you were doing, so it was no problem for me to target my clients' ideal prospect. To make a long story short, we ran the campaign and brought in over $150,000 in cash, and they were as happy as any of my other clients.

In the 1990s, MMC® really dominated health-club marketing. I was advertising in most of the industry's trade magazines to keep the brand out there, as well as mailing out postcards twice a month to every club in the nation. We spent a fortune on advertisement, which paid off because we were doing a ton of business, and by and large, the clubs that wanted to grow their businesses called MMC®.

In the 1990s, several publications asked me to write some articles for their readers, which I was happy to do. It was a win-win, because the publications gave real value to their readers, and I got MMC®'s brand out to all of the clubs that subscribed. In 1999, a staff member from IHRSA (International Health, Racquet, and Sportsclub Association) asked me to be a guest speaker at the health-club convention in Orlando, Florida. I had previously written an article for *CBI* (*Club Business International*) magazine called

"Sales Specifics," and they received so much positive feedback they wanted me to speak on the subject of sales at the their convention. I accepted and invited the club owner from the South Carolina club to come down, as well as a friend of mine who owned a club in South Beach, Florida, that MMC® had done a promotion for, so the two club owners and myself could get a round of golf in and check out the convention before I was to speak.

Once my friends and I got to the hotel, I wanted to prepare for my talk, so I told my friends to go on and golf without me. This speaking engagement was a big deal for me, and I didn't want to let down the people at IHRSA. During my career thus far, I had done over one thousand training sessions, but this was different. This convention was in a big hall, and the place was going to be packed. I knew my material like the back of my hand. I didn't need notes, index cards, or a teleprompter, which I think at the time, concerned the event manager a little.

The following day was the seminar, and I was ready. I spoke on locking up relationships with prospects. I taught the convention attendees how to field informational calls, set up appointments, conduct interviews, tour guests, close sales, and get buddy referrals. The crowd was into it, and most attendees had never known there were actually systems to this process. IHRSA had one of their representatives audit the seminar, and after I was finished, he came up to me and expressed his pleasure with the results and turnout. After a couple of weeks, I received a package in the mail from IHRSA with report cards the participants had filled out. Every card was graded as excellent, and people had written their thoughts about the seminar. I was so happy because I knew I helped so many people that day, and hopefully, they went back to their clubs and implemented just some of what they had learned and became more successful as a result. I was meant to change the industry. It is one of my life's purposes to grow the health-and-fitness industry and make health and fitness affordable for all Americans.

CHAPTER 9

BE CAREFUL WHAT YOU WISH FOR

Within five years, I was up to partnering with about fifty clubs per year. I was rockin', but the business was taking its toll on me. I was traveling to visit prospects through the week and traveling to give sales-training workshops for the new clients on weekends. I was starting to earn a lot of money, but it was all going out for research, market analyses, competitive overviews, consumer profiling systems and data, mailing list compilations, advertising, travel expenses, and general operational costs. I was busting my butt, never staying in one place for more than a couple of days, and I had absolutely nothing to show for it other than a car with over two hundred thousand miles on the odometer. I was sick of the road, and I was operating at maximum capacity because of all of the traveling. I was getting to the point where if I saw one more hotel room, one more fast-food restaurant, one more rental car, or one more airport, I was going to scream!

I desperately needed a change, but I was building a company and wanted to keep growing MMC®. I needed to clone myself because I couldn't see how I could possibly work with more than fifty clubs per year. I needed to leverage my time so I could get off the road and be innovative and creative to grow the company. I wanted to revolutionize the health-club industry, but I couldn't do it as a one-man band. So, I started asking myself questions, starting with, how can I grow MMC® while minimizing my travel? As I told you earlier, if you ask yourself the right questions, you'll get answers. Just make sure you really know what you want, because if you ask the wrong questions, your answers may come back to haunt you. So, my mind delivered four answers to my question: hire salespeople, bring on independent contractors, sell license agreements, or franchise MMC®.

Hiring salespeople just wasn't an option because while living in hotels, I met a lot of on-the-road salesmen and immediately knew the companies footing their expenses were getting hosed big time. They ate expensive meals, drank all night in strip clubs, brought prostitutes back to their hotel rooms, slept in late, and went to their meetings hungover. I had no interest in babysitting salespeople. Independent contractors (ICs) were an option because they would be responsible for their own expenses and would receive commissions on the campaigns they sold, which was how I was compensated my entire adult life—on performance. My challenge with this was I had seen how many ICs went through the revolving doors at both of the previous promotion companies where I had worked. The time spent on training them was ridiculous as well as costly; then after the company spent its money, time, and other resources training them, the ICs went out and tried to compete against their bosses with their bosses' product. My other options were to either sell licenses or franchise MMC®. This way, whomever was representing MMC® would be self-funded and have a vested interest in the success of his or her territory or business (a.k.a. have skin in the game).

I decided to franchise MMC®. My biggest fear was if I brought people into the company, even if they had skin in the game, they would try to take shortcuts which would inevitably devalue the brand, so I really only wanted to offer glorified sales positions and prevent the franchisees from being involved with the behind-the-scenes operations kind of like McDonalds; the corporate office puts it all together and the franchisee just sells the readymade product. After all, MMC® is Chuck Thompson. So, just as in everything I do, I immersed myself into the process of becoming a franchisor.

I hired a franchise consultant to write the uniform franchise offering circular (UFOC) while I was on the road, still selling and running my Cash campaign for clients. The process of building a franchise company in the mid-1990s was extremely expensive and time-consuming. I had to hire several different attorneys specializing in various fields, such as copyright law, trademark law, franchise law, and so on. While all of this was going on, I started thinking; do I really want to have fifty salespeople on the road (one in every state)? Am I going to be able or willing to manage that many people? Is there even enough business to justify that many franchisees? By the time all of the paperwork was done and it was time to register with the states, I had changed my mind. I just wasn't prepared for all of those unknowns, and with that many people, there would definitely be damage done to the product and the MMC® brand. So, I put my stacks of UFOCs on the bookshelves behind my desk in my office, and that is where they died. I also ate more than $100,000 I had invested up to that point. Taking on the role of an entrepreneur sometimes includes taking responsibility for really bad ideas, but you can't worry about the time and money you invested; you must be able to stay focused, be brave, and keep moving forward. If you don't feel you are making the correct decision, you must have the strength to walk away and chalk the investment up as tuition paid for the education.

While I was focused on coming up with a better plan of getting representatives to leverage my time and grow the company, I got a call from a club owner up in Massachusetts. The owner asked whether I could fly up and see him. After doing my homework, I knew his club would do big numbers, so I called him back and set up a meeting. As I was preparing for the trip, I remembered this lady I had met on a flight a while back who gave me her card and told me to look her up if I was ever in Boston. I found the card in my Rolodex (pre-smartphones) and gave her a call. She was pleasantly surprised to hear I was flying up and told me not to rent a car; she would pick me up at the airport and take me to my meeting, afterwards we could go to dinner. This trip was looking better and better every minute.

This lady was really pretty and dressed very well. I have a thing for women who actually wear dresses (I love feminine women), and this lady was very easy on the eyes, with a bangin' body. In the mid-1990s, I was a preferred flyer with a major airline, which came with the perk of being upgraded to first class. Since I was unable to book a direct flight, there were a couple of stops. Every time we landed and took off, she passed by my seat when reboarding the plane, and I was unable able to take my eyes off her gorgeous tiny round athletic gluteus maximus muscle, no matter how hard I tried. This was one trip to Boston I was looking forward to.

I arrived at the airport, and there she was, just as beautiful and sexy as I remembered. We embraced as though we were old friends, said our hellos, and headed to the parking lot. As we rounded the corner, this old, beat-up piece-of-shit tin can caught my eye among all of the beautiful shiny new cars, and I laughed and jokingly thought, I hope she is not driving that damn thing. The lot was packed with nice cars, and there sat this rust bucket on wheels. But as we walked, we kept getting closer and closer to that damn car, and then, my worst fear materialized as she pulled her keys from her purse to unlock the door. I had died and gone to junkyard hell! I am sure she saw the horror in my face; I felt as though I were having an out-of-body experience and looking down on that nightmare. The worst thing was I didn't have enough time to go back inside the airport to rent a car and still make my appointment on time. I had to think and think fast.

Every romantic thought about the evening I had planned for us had completely vanished from my mind, and I went straight into—what the hell am I going to do mode. As she drove, I tried to stay calm and not panic. I didn't want to offend her, because even though her car was the cause of my temporary insanity, I still wanted to start a friendship with her. Had I seen this car any other time, I wouldn't have given it a second thought other than, damn, this girl needs a boyfriend like me who can take better care of her. I am attracted to women for their femininity, not their material possessions or status in life. But at that moment my mind was focused on business and what would be my first impression on the club owner. I had done my due diligence before coming up to Massachusetts; this club was going to bring in at least $300,000 for the owner and about $60,000 for MMC®, and the last thing I could do was have my first impression be in this two-dollar rent-a-wreck. The expression "you never get a second chance at a first impression" is so true. I had to fix this and fix it fast.

On our way to the club, we passed hotel after hotel, and it gave me an idea. I looked at her and said, "If you don't mind, I would like to check in somewhere to freshen up before my meeting." I asked her to pull into a Holiday Inn that was near the club. I checked in, and we went to the room. I showered, got dressed and told her since we had the room for the night, she should just relax and order room service instead of waiting for me in the car. I would go to my meeting alone if she was OK with me driving her car. (Lord only knows why she would have objected; if I had wrecked it, it would have only been an improvement.) She agreed, and I left for my meeting.

My plan was to park the car at a nearby store or business and walk to the club, but oh no, it couldn't be that easy. As I pulled up in front of the club, there was not one business in sight. I drove in all directions, and the closest place seemed like it was a mile away. My mind started racing again; my only option would be to park way in the back of the club, pray no one would see me, get out of the "car," and then walk around to the front door, which is exactly what I did.

I got inside, and it was a nice club. I thought to myself, this club is going to do very well. The owner came up and greeted me, introducing himself, and proceeded to tour me around the club. This club was awesome and had all the amenities and potential to be an enormously successful club. I was thinking, maybe my projections were too conservative. One thing I learned early on in sales is to always underpromise and overdeliver, so even though I thought my projections may have been low, I kept my mouth shut. We ended the tour upstairs and then went into his office. Son of a b——! Right behind his desk was a big picture window looking out over the back parking lot. I couldn't believe this shit. Please, God, tell me he didn't see me park that f——ing thing.

We sat down, and I got right into the presentation, trying not to look out the window. After a few minutes, he stopped me and said, "Chuck, I already know all about MMC® and the campaign. I am ready to get started." My jaw dropped and hit the floor. I immediately knew there was no way he had seen me drive up in that piece of crap, or else he had to be the most desperate club owner in the world, because no club owner in his or her right mind would ever believe someone driving that junker would be able to raise $300,000 in cash in a lifetime much less in just sixty days. This owner said all he needed to know was how fast we could start. I said, "I'll have it launched within seven days, and you'll be collecting revenue within eight days." He signed the agreement and walked me to the front door. As soon as I was out of sight, I bolted back to the rust bucket so I could be in it before he could get upstairs and into his office. I jumped in and drove like a bat out of hell straight back to the hotel.

I launched that club's campaign within a few days, and the campaign immediately took off. We brought in around $50,000 the first week. The owner was calling me every day in jubilation and amazement. Back then, businesses didn't do bank wire transfers as often as we do today, so the clubs were required to FedEx MMC®'s commission check overnight on Monday for Tuesday's delivery. The very first check I received from the owner ($10,000) bounced like a rubber ball (due to insufficient funds); I couldn't believe it. I had just brought in $50,000 in cash for him the week before and was on our way to an additional $50,000 the second week, and he didn't have $10,000 to pay me. He made every excuse you could think of, and even though I knew he was lying, I still wanted to believe him, because he was so convincing and likable. A few days later, the check went through, and we got our money. The rest of the campaign went off without a hitch, and we brought in over $400,000 in cash in less than sixty days.

Toward the end of the campaign, he asked me whether he could come to work for me. My first thought was, are you kidding me? Here was a guy who wrote me one of only two bad checks I had ever received from a client, and now, he wanted to represent MMC®. Fortunately for him, I knew club owners would love to work with this guy because he came across as a well-dressed, well-polished, well-educated, well-groomed, likable guy with the right pedigree. This guy drove the right car and lived in the right house; he really looked and acted the part of a successful club owner. You would think he was the most successful club owner in the world when listening to his stories about his house at the beach, his weekends on the Cape, his ski vacations in Vermont, his golf trips in Florida, and so on.

It is important to know what to look for when hiring a salesperson and then to expand on that search to find a salesperson who can live on the road. Being on the road takes a special breed of person, and it is extremely hard to find people who possess the sales skills who are also well educated, well spoken, well dressed, articulate, immune to rejection, willing to be away from their families for days or weeks at a time, and so on. Salespeople are normally not saddled with the stereotype of having great morals and values like integrity, honesty, honor, and credibility (notice I didn't say "professional" salespeople). Most natural born "salespeople" aren't known to be innovators or have the ability to pay attention to details either. On-the-road salespeople are special in their own way, but once in a great while, you'll find a diamond in the rough, and I was praying this natural born "salesman" was an ole chunk of coal that could be polished into a diamond.

I needed someone I could program with my presentation, someone that could go on the road and visit clubs, freeing me up to be more innovative and creative and to grow MMC®. Of course, this was before the Internet's global acceptance as a tool for conducting business; otherwise, I would have simply done what I do now—put my presentations on video and upload them on our website and YouTube—which keeps MMC®'s message consistent while minimizing the risk of damage to our brand.

In life, and moreover in business, timing is everything, and this natural born "salesman" entered my life at exactly the right time. I wanted help so badly I started rationalizing how he could be just a mouthpiece, and since he had nothing to do with the campaign and was simply in the role of intermediary, he could be contained for the most part. I had already witnessed his natural talent for regurgitating every word I spoke back to me in the same conversation when I did his initial training for his health club in Massachusetts, so I knew he could be programmed. He had come up in the health-club business as a membership salesman; he knew the language of the industry; and he looked the part and knew the health-club business. He also knew MMC®'s Cash campaign from the owner's perspective since we had launched the campaign in his club, so he could relate well to other owners. All I had to do was teach him how to sell the campaign, and with his natural ability to convince people, it would be an easy job for him. So, I decided to give him a try.

The natural born "salesman" lived in New England, so I assigned him to the Northeast, which consisted of about eight states. I had him set up some appointments for us, so I flew up for a week to sell some clubs for him in his new territory. By the end of a week, I had sold a couple of club owners on the Cash campaign. He took to the sales presentation like a duck takes to water. Over dinner each night, he would recite back to me what I had discussed with the owners that day in our meetings. I was impressed and knew he would do very well if he just asserted himself. Being successful in the business of professional sales takes hard work; yes, you can con your way through life with the right look and a gifted tongue, but you will never be truly successful. No matter what, you have to have the drive and determination, study the craft, be willing to work hard, and put in the time. Unfortunately, most natural born "salespeople" are allergic to hard work.

After a couple of years I started noticing a pattern developing with this salesman; he would sell enough clubs to earn around $100,000 or so in commissions, but then he would just disappear. I'd try to call him, and he would give me some lame excuse as to why he wasn't selling, but I knew the truth: he had hit his plateau. Some people are like that. It's like they have thermostats built inside of them, and when they reach certain income levels, they just shut down. For some reason, they don't feel they should earn more, can't imagine earning more, or don't feel they deserve to earn more, but whatever the reason, this was this guy. MMC® was his dream-come-true job because all he had to do was sell club owners on MMC®'s Cash campaign, and my team took over and did everything behind the scenes. He simply handed a finished product each week to his clients and collected a check.

There are two schools of thought in business when it comes to getting your employees to perform: pain and pleasure (a.k.a. the carrot and stick). I like using the mule-and-cart metaphor to illustrate this point. You can motivate mules to pull a cart with carrots (pleasure) or with sticks (pain). Pain is an instant motivator, but it is a short-term tool because once you stop delivering the pain (whipping the mule), he stops pulling the cart. Pleasure, on the other hand, can be a long-term tool but is a much slower process. The trick is to get the carrot out far enough to where the mule can smell the carrot but not close enough to where he can eat the carrot, so he'll keep pulling the cart trying to get to the carrot. I screwed up because I rewarded my "salesman" with not only one carrot but thousands of carrots after he had pulled the cart only a couple of feet; he was so full from one meal it took him weeks before he ever thought about another carrot. Unknowingly, I turned my "salesman" into a hibernating bear. My heart was in the right place because I wanted to show people who "worked" with me they had bright futures ahead if they just worked, and I was willing to reward them well to prove my commitment to their success.

I have always recruited people for specific jobs, jobs they love and possess the skill set to perform. This "salesman" was really just a natural born bullshitter, and that's why I made sure he stayed in sales. I did my best to accept him as he was, and since I knew him well after working with him for a few years, I made it a point to limit his access to clients' campaigns and kept him in an intermediary position.

Within a few months of the "salesman" coming on board with MMC®, I started seeing the "salesman's" true colors and noticed he had a skewed view of the truth. The reason why his first check to MMC® bounced was because his business was completely under water and his creditors were about to seize everything he owned. He paid them with the initial cash to buy some more time. The "salesman" just didn't have the moral compass or work ethic to run a health club and eventually lost the business anyway, which is why he was so set on working with MMC®. No one (including me in the beginning) would ever think for a minute this guy's entire life was nothing but smoke and mirrors.

So, I bet you are thinking by now, Chuck, you seemed like an intelligent guy up to this point, but now you sound like an idiot for keeping this guy on as a "salesman". It's true, he was a pain in the behind sometimes, but only once every year or so would I have to put out a fire, and it affected only MMC® and never a client. Besides, I was always able to fix what he screwed up as long as it was brought to my attention. Most of the time, people loved him. He was an extremely likable guy if you didn't really know him. If you had a drink or dinner with him, you would love the guy, and most of our clients did. I would call some of his clubs just to introduce myself, and they would say nothing but great things about him. He was the perfect front man; while my team wrote the music, played the instruments, and I conducted the orchestra behind the scenes, the "salesman" sat and held the clients' hands and watched the show. As long as he was saying what I had taught him during presentations and no more or less, he could charm clients and their staff members with his personality. This guy just had the knack to make people comfortable, and since MMC® was running the campaign and pulling the strings behind the scenes, everything went smoothly 99.9 percent of the time.

After a few years, I was getting tired of babysitting him, though, and wanted him out of the company. I tried several times to get the "salesman" to leave on his own, but he didn't want to go, he hung on to MMC® like a tick on a dog, and I have a serious flaw (or character trait)—I'm as loyal as a dog. He lost the rights to his original agreement due to countless breaches several years ago, but I allowed him to stay on as an independent contractor. Finally, in January 2015, I decided not to renew his independent contractor's agreement and to cut all ties with him.

On February 16, 2016, MMC®'s office received a complaint from a club manager in Massachusetts regarding this "salesman."

The manager informed me one of MMC®'s past representatives convinced the owner to run a second campaign in March 2015 and allegedly representing himself as still being affiliated with MMC®. I was told this natural born "salesman" proposed that during this online promotion, he as the consultant, would collect all of the revenue from the members' and would then send the owners their percentage of the revenue, kind of like the old promotion companies' arrangement with clubs back in the 1980s he had heard me condemn for years. The owner claimed they had been conned and had never received payment. In their attempts to collect, they had received nothing but excuse after excuse for almost a year, and yet, this "salesman" was still deducting payments from their members' bank accounts and credit-card accounts. Since this "salesman" had represented MMC® in the past, we felt it was our responsibility to contact everyone in his previous sales territory and let them know he had not been affiliated with MMC® since January 2015.

MMC® ran a campaign for this Massachusetts club in 2011 and raised more than $125,000 in immediate cash. It was easy to understand how this alleged con had merit to materialize since this club's ownership already had confidence in MMC®'s marketing campaigns and ethics, due to their previous experience with MMC®. This "salesman" was the club's contact person, so it was easy for the club owner to associate trust to the "salesman" and therefore be easily convinced by his future representations of a new campaign (false or otherwise).

The term "con man" is derived from the word "confidence." A con man normally gains your confidence (trust) with a scheme where you receive the better part of an exchange and then convinces you to trust him again at a later time, when of course you get the short end of the stick, and it is normally shoved up your butt. The hardest part of a con is gaining the confidence of the mark (victim), but once the foundation has been laid, all that is left is the execution of the con. MMC®'s Cash campaign is so successful it was the perfect foundation making it easy for one of our former representatives to use its previous success, as well as MMC®'s good name, to gain the trust and have confidence of one of our past clients.

When we received this call, our team went straight to work on finding this "salesman" for our past client to assist them in retrieving their funds, and in the process, our team found that this guy had even built a website and literally stole every word on his site from MMC®'s website. He did not have one original thought, not one. He even had the balls to take eighteen of MMC®'s clients' testimonials and change the company name from MMC® to his new company's name. I had this guy by the balls; he was guilty of endless counts of corporate theft, copyright infringement and a host of other criminal acts, but the stupidest, most idiotic thing he ever did was to sign every business agreement personally with MMC® over the years, which meant I could not only sue his company but I could also tie up every asset he and his wife had accumulated over their adult lives since he was now personally liable for his actions and could not hide behind a company for protection. But I'm not that kind of guy. I'm not a man who sues; in twenty-five years of being in business, I have never sued anyone, nor have I ever been sued. I hate people like that. "I'm going to sue you" is code for "I'm a loser and want something for nothing." People who sue don't want to be responsible for their own actions or inactions.

I had to pay the price for going against my own values by letting this guy into my life and company, so I had to take responsibility for my own mistake. I believe in karma (what goes around comes around—you get back what you put out), and this "salesman" will get his karma.

Over the next several months, my office received half a dozen complaints about this "salesman" and his con game. He had contacted several of MMC®'s previous clients, trying to sell them on his new promotion. One club called and informed us the "salesman" was claiming to do an online e-mail campaign, using, of course, the only thing he knew—MMC®'s intellectual property and materials.

When someone comes to you claiming he or she will buy or sell you an e-mail list, get as far away from him or her as fast as possible. As I have stated earlier, e-mails are opt-in-only lists. It is unethical to buy e-mail lists, and using them can kill your online presence, and in some cases, get you slapped with a hefty fine or imprisoned. This "salesman" knew all of this from working with MMC® and had heard me condemning the practice numerous times when club owners requested us to buy an e-mail list for their club. He claimed he was buying the e-mail list for $4,200 and sending out the purchased e-mails along with the e-mails from the club's e-mail list. This is a common con known in the digital world. What he really did was only send out e-mails to the club's existing list. He not only collected thousands in ill-gotten commissions but also billed the club for two nonexistent e-mail lists totaling $8,400. This "salesman" allegedly conned the owner out of about $20,000. This was a very easy con for him not only because he used MMC®'s previous campaign as the foundation of his con but because he was also able to capitalize on these owners' hunger for cheap e-mail marketing. As I said earlier, owners hear about these cheap marketing campaigns, and in attempts to save a nickel, they throw away a dollar.

Out of about six complaints one club really stood out because during our investigation, my team discovered the past client actually had been informed this guy was no longer with MMC® in the middle of his "e-mail" campaign (scam) but the club owner liked working with the "salesman" so much he chose to continue working with him anyway. When I called the owner after this truth was uncovered, the owner confirmed my team's discovery and said he couldn't help himself because the "salesman" was so believable and likable. This is one of the many problems with having representatives. People, including customers, like people like themselves and get blinded by their personal relationships. The worst thing was this club brought in $316,000 in the first half of the MMC® Cash campaign that the club owner originally ran with MMC® a year before. He stopped after only two mail drops because he was afraid his club would be too busy. The following year, after the "salesman" had been terminated by MMC®, the owner called the "salesman" on his mobile, thinking he was still with MMC® and told him he wanted to relaunch the campaign because he still had plenty of room for more members (which is exactly what we had told him the previous year). The "salesman" told the owner it was better to do an e-mail campaign instead of finishing the direct-mail campaign because it was much cheaper than direct mail—which was a lie, of course. This owner still had thirty-five thousand pieces of mail sitting in the warehouse, already paid for. All he had to pay was the postage and handling, and he could have earned another $300,000 or more in immediate cash and another $300,000 plus per year for the next two years—he lost a minimum of $900,000 all because he *liked* the "salesman" even when he knew the "salesman" had left MMC®, stolen our property, lied about the direct mail, gave a million off-the-wall excuses as to why the "new" campaign was failing, and had even lied to the club owner about his status with MMC®. Instead of making a million dollars in ninety days with MMC®, he spent six months chasing a criminal for his stolen $20,000.

The owner should have picked up the phone and called MMC®'s home office the minute things started sounding shady and the excuses started (MMC® never makes excuses—our dog has never eaten our homework), but to his detriment, he made a conscious decision to continue to believe the "salesman" even after catching him in numerous lies—karma.

Over twenty-five years, MMC® has had several representatives, and luckily, this was only the second ex-rep who had done anything criminal like this. One other time, many years ago, one of our ICs was terminated, went to a previous client, got her to pay him a $2,500 advance for a new campaign he was peddling, and then, skipped town. Once my team was informed, just as we did in all of the above case we did everything possible to help the club get their money back. This ex-rep had been with MMC® only a few short months and had worked with only two clubs, so he was easily contained. Other than those two incidents, we have never heard of any other theft or fraud from club owners concerning any of our other ex-ICs. I am not saying some guys didn't steal a few of our ideas and our sales presentation trying to start their own companies—that happens every couple of years or so—but their efforts always fail due to their ignorance of the total picture. They have the sales presentation down because that, and only that, is what we taught them, but when the rubber meets the road, they always crash and burn.

Because of this ex-representative (the "salesman"), we at MMC® had to make drastic changes in the way we do business. We no longer have outside reps or ICs, other than one who has been with us for over ten years. Other than him, all of our reps now are either employed by MMC® or have left the company. There are no more lone wolves running wild throughout the United States that we know of, but please let us know if you run into one. All of MMC®'s presentations are now on video and uploaded on our website (healthclubmarketingmmc.com) for our prospects to view at their leisure. If a customer wants to speak to one of our representatives, all he or she has to do is call our office at 904-217-3762 (toll-free 877-620-8135) or e-mail me at chuck@mmctoday.com.

The biggest and greatest threat to the health-club industry as a whole is not criminals like this "salesman", its copycats. Criminals always get caught and worst-case scenario may affect a dozen health clubs, whereas copycats are far more dangerous because their thievery spreads like a virus throughout the industry, killing every business in its path. Unfortunately, I see this way too often in the health-club industry. How many times have you designed a great marketing plan only to have your competitor launch an identical campaign within just a few months of yours, and soon after, every health club within sixty miles is running your campaign?

When all of the clubs in your area are running exactly the same offer, targeting the same segment of prospects and the same demographics, with the same price-point, the piece of the pie for each club just gets smaller and smaller. The first club to be seated at the table always gets the largest piece, and the last club to be seated is left with just the crumbs. The main reason each consecutive club gets a smaller slice is not because all of the prospects are gone out of the market; it's because the quality of the campaign is deteriorating with each copy. Think about it logically; each health club is in a different geographical area, and since most health clubs pull from at least a five-mile radius, each club is going to have some (if not the largest) portion of its population that does not overlap with the other clubs in the area running the same campaign, leaving a large portion of the population untouched, which would lead you to believe the offer should still pull well.

Wrong! It is not that the offer stops pulling; it is that the details of the campaign have been diminishing from club to club. This is just like when you photocopy something over and over; it gets less visible unless you change the ink cartridge. The same applies when someone is copying a promotional offer; it gets weaker and weaker each time it is copied. This is because each club gets further and further away from the original design and implementation. In short, too many cooks in the kitchen are going to spoil the stew.

Forget what your neighbor is doing because more than likely, he or she is doing what his or her neighbor did, and they are both doing it wrong. Copying your competitor's marketing or business model is a recipe for disaster. Growing a business is similar to playing chess; you must be thinking at least three moves in advance of your competitor; not following behind him. If you continue to play the copying game or follow the leader—you will always be behind in the game.

I'll use MMC®'s Cash campaign as an example: When competitors of clubs partnering with MMC® see our Cash campaign being launched for our client's club, inevitably one or two of the competitors will try and copy the campaign within a few months because no matter how great their club is—they will definitely feel the pain of MMC®'s Cash campaign. The competitor assumes (ass-u-me, is when you make an *ass* of *you* and *me*) they know everything there is to know about the campaign when all they know is the price-point and what they heard through the grapevine either from their members or a colleague in the industry. Because of their ignorance and desperation, they launch the campaign in their club ruining their business and market forever, because all they have done is give a cheap membership to health-and-fitness-conscious consumers who would have paid the club's published rates.

But wait, the situation gets even worse because now another competitor on the other side of their market sees the first competitor running the campaign and copies what he or she can, which is now down to about 2 percent of the original campaign because the first competitor cut corners to save money and implemented only half of what he or she copied. By the time the fifth club copies the abbreviated version of the Cash campaign all that is left of the original campaign is the price-point. It is this perversion of MMC®'s Cash campaign (focusing solely on the price-point) that is killing the health-club industry.

Under normal circumstances, if a promotion yields three hundred members, you should throw a party and celebrate. Three hundred members from a campaign like MMC®'s Cash campaign is considered a huge flop, because those three hundred members came from your core market. Most media, including social and e-marketing platforms, target your core market and preexisting customers. If you do not incorporate a consumer profiled list based on specific criteria identifying the consumer's spending habits designed to recognize the deconditioned consumer who has purchased within the health or fitness categories within the past twelve months with a message tailored to their psychological needs delivered via personalized direct mail which is put directly in their hands—you're hanging yourself with the little rope you got for free.

When clubs put their ads in newspapers, on the radio, and on social-media platforms, the only people who are paying attention to them are the consumers who are already paying attention and are presently a part of the club's prospect community. There are three important factors novices fail to realize. First, almost every generation gets its news and information from different media and platforms. Second, anyone with a great facility who is willing to drop his or her pants (rates) can easily capture the health-and-fitness segment of the market. Third, the only way to grow a business is to acquire the segments or groups that are not being engaged because these segments actually grow the business as well as the industry. If a club is not tapping into new markets and segments they are just recycling members.

"Cherry pickers" is a term I use to describe those people that target the low-hanging fruit and leave all of the other fruit on the tree. They do exactly the same with prospects. They cherry-pick a promotion, a website, a presentation, a campaign or whatever else they can get their hands on to get the quick and easy information to sell the easiest prospects but because of their greed and lack of innovation, they inevitably leave 80 percent of the fruit on the tree. Talk about leaving money on the table; these "geniuses" are like bank robbers who empty out the tellers' drawers but leave the safe untouched. They naively think they are cherry-picking a campaign for the good stuff when all they do is ruin the fruit for themselves as well as everyone else.

One of the other huge mistakes clubs often make is they design a losing package. They either give everything away or don't give enough to make the campaign successful. Finding the right balance between value and investment is paramount to the success of any campaign. It took me years of managing countless campaigns to understand the dynamics of the product well enough to maximize the return while eliminating the downside. Having the ability, or inability, to adjust on the fly can make or break any campaign. After twenty-five years of managing the Cash campaign, our team is still faced with unforeseen challenges from time to time, although nowhere near as many as I faced in the first five years after launching my first campaign. A campaign of this magnitude consumes hours upon hours of our staff's time, and in my experience, most owners and managers don't have extra staff or extra time.

Most owners, as well as their staff members, are already wearing too many hats, yet most owners want to saddle their staff with this enormous responsibility of growing the club. It is my bet that you, the owner, are constantly disappointed with the performance of your club. A successful campaign demands hours and hours from personnel to monitor social media, gather data, conduct surveys, run competitive overviews, and so on and even more importantly, each step, task and phase are all time sensitive. If you are having a hard time just getting your staff to show up to work on time or to remember to have guests sign in at the front desk or get the contact information form an information call or even the simplest of tasks like have every member check in at the front desk—how on earth are they going to manage a million-dollar marketing campaign, especially when they don't have the materials, system, resources, experience, or necessary data.

Any given campaign launched by MMC® has a minimum of thirty people's fingerprints on it. MMC®'s success fee is only 20 percent of the cash collected from the gross sales collected at the point of sale, which works out to be less than 4 percent of the total revenue (immediate cash and back-end revenue) brought in by MMC®. This is not a get-rich-quick scheme. But only people who study (not steal) would know this.

There is an old saying in the legal world: "A man who is his own lawyer has a fool for a client and an idiot for an attorney." This holds true for a health-club owner trying to run a million-dollar campaign without the proper training, tools, experience and data; or even worse, letting an employee run it that has no skin in the game. Forget for a minute that I am the one saying this, and think logically for a second. If you own a club, you get one shot at running a campaign of this magnitude; if you, your employee, or whoever you hire makes only one mistake (out of hundreds of possible mistakes), you could literally screw up your club's financial future or—even worse—bankrupt the business.

I am a firm believer in people asking themselves good questions. Ask yourself this: Have you or your staff ever launched a million-dollar campaign? I am absolutely sure the answer is no. Then why on earth would you think in your wildest imagination you or your staff would be qualified to launch and manage MMC®'s Cash campaign? Even with all of the information I have shared with you in this book of things to do and examples of things not to do, you have less than 20 percent of what goes into one of our campaigns and absolutely none of the data, profile or experience yet you know a thousand times more than these "geniuses" who try to copy it. I am writing this book for the same reason I built an educational website—so you can learn how to develop your *own* marketing and sales programs. I am just using my MMC®'s Cash campaign as an example so you can see how this entire system came together and revolutionized an entire industry to inspire you to do the same for your *own* product or service. This book is meant to educate and inspire you to bring value and innovation to the industry.

My biggest grievance with people copying MMC®'s price-point other than it is killing the health-club industry is that it does horrific damage to MMC®'s brand. When club owners and industry people see a club run a campaign with a lower barrier-to-entry they automatically assume the club partnered with MMC® whether they had or not. Unfortunately, the majority of these health clubs that copy our campaign go out of business because they ruin their own market and destroy their club's brand. Everybody then starts to link the closure to MMC®, and they don't realize we had nothing to do with the club's promotion or closure—we, too, are victims.

MMC®'s clients don't go out of business and our clients' employees don't lose their jobs. There are a number of our club owners who choose to sell their business after partnering with us in a campaign but this is only because the business experiences its greatest net worth after MMC® closes out our Cash campaign. Our campaigns are designed to penetrate new markets and segments not cannibalize current ones. When club owners target their core customers, they have nowhere to turn other than bankruptcy, but when they partner with MMC®, the possibilities of growth are endless.

Some health-club marketing companies are plagued with laziness, lack of innovation and complacency. Let me share just a couple of the most recent instances with you to shine some light on this statement. One day, MMC®'s research team was surfing the net and found a description for one of our videos copied and pasted onto a competitor's video that was uploaded on YouTube. Unfortunately, that wasn't the worst part. The worst part was the competitor even copied MMC®'s name and left it with the description of *their* video. This same competitor, who is legendary for plagiarism, got a copy of our free download on locking up relationships off of our website and built a membership site where he is selling the information to club owners for a premium. When my staff showed me the membership site, I was flabbergasted because it was blatantly obvious he had downloaded all of the information for free from MMC®'s site and was even too lazy to change most of the wording. He even copied Einstein's definition of insanity, which has been on our site for decades. These frauds don't have one original thought or idea, yet they con owners into believing they are authorities on the subjects of sales and marketing.

Another example is a company that recently copied the language of one of our videos about copycats and put it on their site. They did this to deflect suspicion, but it was obvious they frequently troll our site for our talking points and just rewrite sound bites and post them on their site to pass them off as original content. They are too ignorant to go into any detail because they don't know the material behind the talking points they copied, but the message sounds great because it is MMC®'s message. The only valuable content on their website is what they cherry-pick from MMC®'s site. Our team at MMC® built our website as an informational and educational research hub for club owners, but these impotent copycats follow us closer than a stray cat. Their claim to fame is their company has over thirty years of experience in the industry. When a business person references longevity, it should be the experience of the owner or the longevity of the company, not the accumulated experience of several partners and employees. I have been in the membership, marketing, and *professional*-sales business since 1982; that's thirty-five years of actual real-time experience. It is misleading and a false representation if you advertise thirty years of experience, because five people in your company each have six years in the industry. It's impossible to say you have thirty years of experience in the health-club industry when you are only thirty or forty years old.

Another thing that drives me nuts is when I read an excerpt from someone's book or site claiming he or she has sold millions of memberships or has made millions of dollars selling health-club memberships, yet the person is in his or her mid-thirties and has only operated a handful of clubs. It is so easy to prove he or she is full of crap, because numbers don't lie, and if you just run the numbers, you'll see the impossibility of their claims. I read and hear hyperbole like this all of the time on websites and in books; it's a complete falsehood. "Marketers" like these BS artists have a casual relationship with the truth and should be run out of the health-club industry.

"Imitation is the sincerest form of flattery," and we at MMC® are truly flattered by those who try to copy or imitate us, but it is health-club owners as well as the industry we worry about the most, because although the imitators may sound like us, they are nothing like us at all. MMC® is celebrating its twenty-fifth anniversary in business. We have launched more than seven hundred successful campaigns since 1991. We have worked with over five hundred health clubs and over two hundred golf courses. We have sold over 750,000 memberships. We have raised over $175 million in up-front cash and over $400 million in back-end revenue for a total of over $575 million in revenue for our partnering clubs and clients.

Before I open MMC® in 1991, I had worked with over 250 health clubs either as an employee, independent contractor for a promotion company, consultant, or under the CTC brand. In that period of almost a decade, I sold or was directly responsible for selling more than 250,000 memberships representing more than one hundred clubs. In total I have been responsible for more than one million memberships and over a half billion dollars in revenue. These numbers are not arbitrary—these numbers are a fact!

MMC® doesn't take up-front fees; our campaigns are completely self-funding; there is absolutely no risk when running our campaigns; we are driven by up-to-date data; we are a performance-based company (which means we get paid only on our performance and success); we really do put our money where our mouths are, because we pay all of our own expenses before, during, and after the campaign; and our campaigns are completely turnkey. Our personnel perform 99 percent of the work, while the club's staff collects the money and builds relationships with the new members. Our clients deposit all the money into their banks, never into ours. We have a 100 percent satisfaction guarantee; if our clients are not completely happy with our campaigns, they won't owe us a dime. These are not just words or something we copied from someone else—these are facts built into the DNA of MMC®.

MMC®'s Cash campaign was never meant to be a business model; the marketing concept is to give a club a jump-start by acquiring hundreds, if not thousands of members at one time from untapped segments of the market and convert them into long-term members. Unfortunately, after a lot of club owners ran the Cash campaign, they became addicted to the cash and forgot this campaign was designed as a mulligan (a "do-over" or a second chance) to rejuvenate a club's traffic, revenue, and membership base by balancing out their membership. In no way is it meant to become the price-point of a club or the norm for the entire industry. The long-term strategy is to acquire a surplus of members, continue marketing, while gradually increasing the membership rates as well as the perceived value of the club within the community.

Instead of following through with the long-term strategy, some clubs just continued to run the campaign day after day, changing only what was being offered for $99.00 per year or $9.99 per month—limited memberships, amenities, initiation fees, unlimited three-month tanning programs and so on—to the point where the price-point became the norm, and within ten years, owners all across the United States were scratching their heads, blaming the lower barrier-to-entry concept to the downfall of their businesses as well as the industry as a whole.

Unfortunately, because of all of these copycats and knock-offs, the industry has been saturated with discounted memberships, and by about 2010, you could go anywhere and get a membership for only $9.99 a month or $99 a year. MMC®'s original price-point for our EFT campaign was $9.99 a month, but again, this was for a limited introductory membership, targeting a new segment of the market and was never meant to be sold to the health-conscious consumer. The lower barrier-to-entry was designed only to be used as a hook and never to be run for more than ninety days.

Today, you can get a full club membership for only $9.99 a month or $99 a year in just about any town. This is an absolute travesty. This stupidity is why so many health-club owners are barely getting by. It's not the economic climate, the saturation of health clubs, the housing collapse, or the millennials; it's stupidity, greed and pure laziness. It is the perversion of MMC®'s Cash campaign and the abuse of the $9.99 and $99 hooks that is ruining the health-club industry. I engineered MMC®'s Cash campaign and EFT campaign to grow businesses by engaging and locking up relationships with the deconditioned market, not to cannibalize the health-conscious market.

The goal behind MMC®'s model is to bring in a ton of new members on a one-time introductory rate and immediately start building the perceived value of the club via different marketing campaigns designed to show the community that the club is far more valuable than the previous introductory offer implied; that offer was a one-and-done and will never be offered again. MMC®'s staff even informs the client's community this was a campaign where the club was willing to buy the consumer's loyalty in hopes of building a long-term relationship. I repeat: the most difficult part of growing a membership base is getting prospects through the door. This "lost leader" with a lower barrier-to-entry concept; whether $99.00 per year or $9.99 per month was designed only as a hook to grab the attention of the deconditioned market and get them in the door of the health club.

Owners feared the ninety-nine-dollar promotion so much that it became the model for the industry. The club owners who fear the concept are like the driver of a new sports car who is on an open road and decides to see what the car can do, so he or she accelerates until soon, he or she loses control and wraps the shiny new sports car around a telephone pole. Later, family and friends come to the scene of the accident and look around in bewilderment at how their loved one could have ever hit the pole, because there isn't another pole or anything else around for a mile; there's nothing but wide-open flat land. Drivers hit telephone poles on open roads because that is what they fear worse than anything else at the time; their focus stays locked in on the pole and since it is human nature to steer in the direction of your focus, the driver steers straight into the pole. This is the perfect metaphor for the health-club industry. Most owners were so afraid of the ninety-nine-dollar promotion that they never embraced it or used the tool properly. They stuck their toes in the water a little and tried to redesign the campaign to fit their needs, but they forgot the most basic rule in business: if it ain't broke, don't fix it.

Over the years, I have been concerned about how I would come across if I wrote articles or spoke out on the subject of how and why the industry is dying a slow death. I shied away from doing so until now because I didn't want to appear to be a bitter employer or as if I were just trying to bash my competition—neither of which is true in the least. This is in no way a condemnation of my competitors because I am all for competition. I'm an athlete and I welcome strong competition because it allows me to compare the superiority of my campaigns to those of others. Anyone taking a dollar out of your field of expertise is considered competition, but that's OK. Competition has never hurt MMC®, because let's face it: there are approximately thirty-five thousand health-club-related membership based businesses in the United States alone. There is plenty of business to be *earned* by all *legitimate* marketing companies. I believe in competition, but I believe in competing with individuals or companies who compete on their own merits. I believe in competing in a way that is going to benefit the industry as a whole and will make all of us working in this industry stronger and wiser. Conmen, plagiarist, cherry pickers, copycats and hackers don't make anything better or bring anything of value to the table; instead they are destroying the industry by running health-club businesses into the ground.

The fact is, it is the copycats, conmen, hackers (a golf term for someone who just hacks at the ball with absolutely no skill), and cherry pickers who are responsible for making it nearly impossible to earn a good living owning a health club today. These guys put more clubs out of business because of their incompetence than any recession or depression ever could. They have killed the industry as a whole. Think about it: for every campaign MMC® has launched, the price-point was copied at least ten times (sometimes twenty or more). Then, add in the clubs that just copied the hook for their own promotions: aerobics, tanning, or personal-training sessions. These knock-offs spread throughout the industry like a virus, killing clubs along the way. It is absolutely absurd to sell an unrestricted membership to health-and-fitness-conscious consumers for $99.00 per year or $9.99 per month. These numbers are *hooks*, nothing more. Operating a health club is expensive, and operating a club properly by offering unparalleled customer service is even more expensive.

Let's face it, the positives about the health-club industry are readily available, and everyone in the business is ready to sing its praises and has done so in thousands of books. Unfortunately, it is not the great things about the industry that need to be addressed if the industry is going to get the "good ole days" back. The industry is full of yes-men; it needs solutions, not the same old, same old. Someone must be willing to address the challenges and provide solutions to grow the industry and health and fitness in general.

I stated in chapter 8, I was born to champion causes, and I have a new cause. I am determined to make owning a health club one of the most profitable businesses in America, and in the world, for that matter. There are more unhealthy consumers than ever before, and it is time health clubs learn how to effectively market their products and services to all demographics, including the deconditioned segment as well as millennials. I am still an advocate for affordable health and fitness, but I am also an advocate for businesses to make respectable profits for providing valuable services. Everyone in the health-club business sells the greatest product on earth, that is, health and fitness, and more and more people need our help as an industry. So, once again, I have a new mulligan for health clubs.

In the next and final chapter, I will lay out a step-by-step marketing strategy and share with you my thoughts and predictions for the health-club industry's future. There is a bright future, and club owners can make respectable livings while still making health and fitness affordable for all Americans.

For all of you who are reading this book who do not own a health club you will learn the greatest marketing strategy in the world for the long-term growth of any business. I am including my five-year growth intuitive for health clubs for you to use as a guide to build your own marketing strategy for your health-and-fitness product or service. Don't focus on the fact that is MMC®'s presentation instead focus on how you can apply the same principles to your own marketing strategy, growth intuitive, and presentation.

CHAPTER 10

UNDERSTANDING THE TASK AT HAND

There are numerous statistics and studies on health and fitness as well as on the health-club industry. Most studies claim approximately 70 percent of Americans are health conscious, yet only 16–20 percent (depending on the study) of the population has committed to a traditional health-club membership or loyalty program at one time or another. However, these customers (16 to 20 percent of the American population) will work out or train somewhere in their local communities and join health clubs near their homes or workplaces at least once in their lives. If you have adequate facilities and strong marketing strategies (tangible or intangible); you will capture your market share. However, I have never believed in market share. I believe in market domination, and in this chapter I am going to guide you through a step-by-step action plan that will give you the tools to dominate your market by locking up relationships with the remaining 50 percent of consumers who are health conscious but have eluded all other marketing efforts and linger in the uncommitted segment. I emphasize the uncommitted 50 percent because any competent marketer with a great product should be able to capture their share of the 16 to 20 percent who are already interested in a health-club membership.

The health-club industry is in the middle of a storm. The facility in your area that is best marketed, educated, prepared, and represented will capture the attention of the 20 percent that is already committed to exercise, and that club will successfully weather the current storm as well as those storms that will inevitably follow. Unfortunately, those who do not embrace the importance of promoting their products to capture market share will pay the ultimate price.

Many health clubs have left the marketplace in the last few years. Theories circulate the country as to why, ranging from too much inventory—too many health clubs and not enough members—to the present economic climate and so on. This plague of closures started years ago, yet this deficit (yes, I believe there is a shortage of health clubs, and we as an industry are losing more and more each year) in inventory has yet to equate to increased revenue or memberships for the survivors, even though there are more consumers pledging their loyalties to health clubs around the United States. Thinning out the herd is not the answer. There is room for all health clubs if they are marketed properly.

By misdiagnosing the problem, we will never be able to fix it. If a doctor misdiagnoses an ailment and prescribes the wrong medicine, the patient will more than likely get worse or even die. The same goes for the health-club industry. If owners keep listening to the narrative being shaped by some of the industry "experts," their businesses are going to continue suffering.

In 2016, there are twice as many people joining health clubs as there were just a couple of decades ago. People are making far better choices when it comes to their health and fitness, and studies as well as statistics show the younger generations (Y, Z, and the millennials) are willing to invest far more when it comes to their health than any of the previous generations. Education and awareness programs have been fueling this surge in health-conscious consumers since the 1980s, but it has only been over the past couple of years that health categories grew faster than indulgent categories. Studies show more than fifty-five million Americans are joining health clubs, yet most health clubs are barely getting by; the math just doesn't add up.

Sixty-five percent of Americans are overweight or obese. More than forty-five million Americans go on diets each year. There are approximately thirty-five thousand membership-based exercise clubs in the United States, which means the average gym, fitness center, health club, athletic club, and so on should have at least fifteen hundred members. If the average membership in the United States is $40 a month, then every club theoretically should be grossing a minimum of $60,000 a month, or $720,000 a year, in membership fees and at least another $280,000 in back-end revenue, bringing the average club's revenue to $1 million per year.

You have heard me say it, and I am saying it again: numbers don't lie. With numbers like these, every health club in America should be making money hand over fist, so why aren't they? It's because they are still running marketing campaigns from the 1990s and marketing to the same segment of health-conscious consumers as their competitors—the health-and-fitness-conscious consumer. Most clubs need as many (or more) uncommitted members as committed members to balance out the membership base. Owners should be thinking in terms of three thousand members (depending on the size of their facilities, but anything over ten thousand square feet would easily qualify for three thousand members), with two thousand coming from the uncommitted segment. The uncommitted segment works out far less often but spends drastically more per visit than the committed segment. The uncommitted segment is where you'll find the real profit margin and growth. When you capture this group, you'll increase your back-end revenue by 50 to 250 percent in addition to a ton of up-front cash.

When faced with hard economic times, a lot of owners and operators think of four ways to increase revenue. The first thought is to raise membership dues on existing members. This is a huge mistake because the fallout of disgruntled members offsets the increased revenue. These members were probably just waiting for a logical excuse to quit anyway, and now you have handed it to them on a silver platter. This plan results in a loss of revenue more often than not. The only way this can work is if you are starting with a surplus of members and are prepared for the inevitable fallout.

Another ill-conceived plan to increase revenue is to get existing members to spend more in the profit centers. This too rarely works since consumers fall into spending patterns and develop buying habits, and it is extremely difficult to change these conditioned routines. Members are conditioned from the point of sale, and if you have not conditioned them to stop at the juice bar to buy a protein shake or a bottle of water, they never will. If you try to condition them a year or two down the road, your efforts may be perceived as greedy by your loyal members. The delicate balance between conditioning and marketing will be important to your long-term growth.

Others believe the only way to survive this economic storm is to cut costs, and they usually start by cutting payroll, which in turn diminishes service, which leads to unsatisfied members, who eventually leave the club. The health-club industry is a service industry. If we want to thrive (not just survive), we must provide unparalleled customer service. Members want to feel like members, as if they belong, are welcome, and are appreciated. Remember it costs six times as much to acquire a new member as it does to keep (service) an existing member, so do the math, and provide the best customer service your budget will allow. No one has ever cut (customer service) his or her way to prosperity.

The best way to raise revenue and thrive in this or any storm is by bringing in new business and conditioning the new members' spending habits at the point of sale. This is exactly what MMC® does; we bring in new business from an untapped segment, immediate cash, and increased revenue from profit centers, which equates to long-term residual income. I have developed proven campaigns that target a group of individuals that 99 percent of all other health clubs and marketing companies have neglected. I have had the luxury of traveling all over the United States and throughout the world, researching and compiling the most current data to develop a marketing strategy and a professional sales-training system designed specifically to support MMC®'s approach to ensure you dominate your market, not just secure market share. MMC® has invested millions of dollars in demographic and market research since 1991, eliminating the guesswork to provide our clients a proven method that works in the real world.

MMC®'s clients don't go out of business, and our clients' workers don't lose their jobs. You may ask why that is. It's because we capture new business from an untapped segment and rebuild old relationships. Whether our customers come from the health-and-fitness conscious or the deconditioned segments, all of our customers have been selected through a thorough profiling criteria based formula to assure the maximum ROI from our marketing efforts at a minimal expense. This is how you grow your health club—not by raising members' dues, not by forcing members to buy unwanted products, and definitely not by cutting customer service.

Like it or not, there is a new norm for the health-club industry. If you own or manage a health club and you want to thrive in the health-club business or, worst-case scenario, simply be financially solvent over the next ten years, you had better suspend your ego for a few minutes and read this chapter with an open mind. The health-club industry has yet to see its hardest hit, but it is coming and coming really soon. I have been predicting trends in the health-club industry since the early 1980s. Each time I have made a prediction, I have been spot-on, but not because I am a Nostradamus wannabe. I am far from a genius either, but I am a lifelong student of marketing, sales, psychology, economics, history, social sciences, and more specifically, professional club membership sales. Here is what the data shows.

First, you must accept the fact that the spending habits of everyday people are what drives the economy—the spending habits of groups or segments, not individuals. Not everyone (as an individual) falls into this matrix, but as a group, people do predictable things at certain stages in their lives. If you want to know the year you are most likely to die, just ask your insurance provider, and after he or she asks you a few lifestyle questions, he or she will be able to give you a very good guess. These demographic realities are all based on data that has been collected and analyzed over decades. Similar data is available for the economy; if you simply know where to look and, more importantly, know how to interpret the data, you can easily see the future as well.

There is an enormous amount of data available that tells us at what age (as a group) Americans are likely to do certain things, make major purchases, and make life-changing decisions. For example, on average, we join the workforce around twenty-two years old; we marry at an average age of twenty-six; we buy our first home at an average age of thirty-one; we buy bigger houses at an average age of thirty-nine; and we are in positions to have our greatest disposable income (what is referred to as our peak spending years) at an average age of forty-six, which is when we tend to buy luxury items—sports cars and boats—travel more frequently, and so on. We tend to continue this spending pattern up to the age of fifty-three, and after that, our spending habits start to drop off dramatically because we then start saving for our retirement. We typically enter retirement at age sixty-three, and once we retire, our spending comes to a halt other than for medical-related expenses. This is not a guess; this is a demographic fact. This data is all over the Internet absolutely free; look it up.

The reason why the United States experienced a great rush in the 1990s is because we were in the middle of the baby boomers' peak spending years. Baby boomers were the largest generation in the history of the United States up to that point, and that is why health clubs experienced massive growth, which inevitably sparked the growth in the construction of new health clubs. Because of the baby boomers entering their peak spending years, health clubs had a huge influx of members. During the 1990s, everyone and their brother were opening health clubs. This is exactly why some of the so-called experts are claiming we have too much inventory today in 2016 and not enough members. This statement is absurd as well as ignorant. There are plenty of prospects out there; the challenge is most club managers and owners are living in the past and are too stubborn and egotistical to accept the reality and change with the times.

Around 2006, the baby-boomer generation completed their spending cycle and started to slow down on spending. By now (2016), the last rush of big spenders has retired, which means their money has now been removed from the economy and has been put into safe, low- to no-risk investments in preparation for their golden years. This is why the health-club industry has never seen an upturn in business since the decline (which really started in 2003), even though most economists say the economy is getting better. By the way, I strongly disagree with that statement as well. It is my belief things will be terrible (much worse than in 2008) for the next decade because there is no other generation that can possibly fill this enormous void in spending over the next decade since the largest generation in history (until the millennial) is retired or dying. Even if I am wrong, the millennials are the generation clubs are going to have to engage and lock up relationships with, and they are the most difficult consumers to date. Millennials won't start hitting their spending cycles for at least a decade, and generation X can't fill that vacuum because baby boomers (a.k.a. the "Me Generation") had far fewer children than previous generations, which equates to far less spending.

I am not trying to guess the future of the club business; I am just stating the facts. In no way is this chapter meant as a warning of Armageddon. Quite the contrary, it is a road map to financial freedom. People always say knowledge is power, but I disagree; a lot of us know what we should do but never do it. Case in point, we all know we should eat healthy, exercise, and get six to eight hours of uninterrupted sleep every night, but do we follow those simple steps to healthier, longer, happier lives? This is of course a rhetorical question because even though we know we should. Instead, action coupled with knowledge is ultimate power.

The great news is the millennial generation is bigger (by almost 15 percent) than the baby-boomer generation, which means in about a decade from now (2016), things will be rockin' again, and everyone (even the uninformed) will be making a fortune. The tip for the future success of clubs is demographics, because the millennial generation is far more diverse than the baby boomers.

The business of owning and marketing a health club has changed, and it will be a decade or more before the industry gets anywhere close to where it was in past decades. If you don't change your antiquated business model and rethink your inadequate marketing, your business will die with the baby boomers. Forget marketing concepts of the past because they won't work with millennials, and do not be conned (convinced) by the false narrative that the only way to engage millennials is via e-marketing, social media, or other platforms of digital marketing. Most millennials change their platforms from year to year, jumping on the latest coolest platforms. Yes, a working knowledge of digital marketing is essential, but first, you must create a model that offers products and services specifically tailored to the buying patterns and spending habits of this generation (not generations of the past); then, and only then, can you decide on the best delivery system to get the message or offer out.

Social-media platforms are changing so fast. First, the hottest platform was Facebook, then Twitter, then Instagram, and then Snapchat, and so on. Targeting millennials is far more difficult than starting a Facebook or Twitter account. Millennials jump platforms like prospective members jump from club to club, looking for the deal of the day. About every two years, there is a new popular platform. The only way to get in the millennial's circle and follow their next step is to get them in your circle first, and they (as a group) will keep you informed of the new trends in social media.

Again, this lack of information is just one more example of everyone missing the boat. Owners, managers and salespeople buy into the BS that saturates the Internet about e-marketing. Social-media marketers want you to believe you need them or you'll never engage millennials. The fact is millennials have to live somewhere, and there is no better media to engage them than a profiled, personalized piece of direct mail. For some reason, the so-called experts out there think you must reinvent the wheel, just as a lot of industry people think they need to reinvent the industry, when that is the furthest from the truth. You do need to update and upgrade your facility over time, but the wheel is the wheel, just as a health club is a health club.

The other day, I was speaking with one of my sons (Chaz), who was totally immersed in his devices and gadgets. I asked him why he was using his computer and iPad at the same time. He replied, "Dad, one is for streaming video, and the other is for gaming." He then informed me his sister (Azha) uses three devices at a single time, because not only is she gaming and streaming videos, but she chats as well. Millennials are the new generation of consumers. If you can get to just a few millennials, and your message resonates with them, you may get lucky and have your message go viral within their circle of friends. But you would be foolish to assume this will happen. You must be well versed in all media and platforms so you're not just hoping for a successful campaign but planting the seeds ensuring a successful campaign.

Another point on digital or e-marketing that needs to be touched on is SEO (search-engine optimization). Understanding SEO is extremely important to maintain an online presence. SEO is the system or strategy used on the Internet to get better rankings with search engines like Google, Yahoo, Bing, and so on. When a prospective member searches online to get information about a health club and you have worked on your SEO, your health club will appear in one or more of the top five results on the first page. The reason you will want this position on the page is because if your site shows up after page 1 of the search results, the percentage of prospects who will see your information will be few if any. There are basically ten spots on the first page, and you want to be number one if at all possible. The search-result statistics change day to day, as do the percentages of views and clicks that you receive by being number one and then number two, three, four, five, and so on. But on average, you are going to get probably 35 percent or better of the clicks if you're number one, and after that, the percentages will go down as low as 3 percent on the first page.

But the most important thing for you to understand when it comes to SEO is that your goal is to be a top-ranked health club within your keyword searches. For example, if you are in Chicago and someone searches for "health clubs in Chicago," you want to be ranked number one with the top search engines. You can accomplish this by adding back links, writing blogs, putting keywords on your website, getting involved with social media, buying a domain name with your town and product in the address, for example, chicagoabchealthclub.com, since prospect are more than likely going to search for Chicago health clubs, and so on. These are all essential tools to help you get better rankings with the major search engines. The key thing is to make sure you provide free education and information on your website. You must also make sure you have new content often to keep the search-engine crawlers coming back to your site. This is one of the reasons why businesses and individuals load up on social media; they want more traffic to their websites so they can get better rankings with the search engines within their niches.

There are numerous mistakes you can make when it comes to your search-engine results. In 2012 and then again in 2014, I had to make a decision to change MMC®'s domain name, which killed our ranking and made us start over from scratch. I decided to move away from using our original domain, healthclubconsultant.com—which I started in 1999 and which was organically ranked number one or two on Google for more than a decade. Of course, this was against the advice of our in-house SEO specialist. But the word "consultant" doesn't define MMC® as a company, because we specialize in the design and implementation of marketing campaigns. Believe me, it was painful to see competitors who started their companies fifteen or twenty years after MMC® jump ahead of us in ranking overnight, especially when at least 20 percent of the content on their websites came from our website. But sometimes, you have to make difficult decisions, and since I knew we were in business for the long haul, I bit the bullet.

Even though most digital platforms do not produce a stunning ROI, the long-term branding of your club, name recognition, brand positioning in the marketplace, list building and so on will pay dividends tenfold throughout your career. You can't major in minor things if you want enormous success. Big numbers are relative; the more contacts you make, the more people you'll help and more money you'll make. So, you must turn over every rock, not just the easy ones, and if you can't afford to hire the experts in those specific fields needed, you must learn a little bit about all of the resources available to get your name, product, or service out into the marketplace.

A major component of running a successful business is ABP (always be prospecting). I believe in guerilla marketing. Advertising is paramount to success; the more you do of it, the more success you will experience. Do it all, and do it always. When it comes to marketing and prospecting, Steady Eddie is the way. Stay consistent with your message, and keep your name in front of your targets. Timing is everything, and this holds especially true in advertising as well. I do strongly believe social media and e-marketing will be mainstream tools for marketing to all generations in another decade so you better start preparing now.

Everyone is depending on you to grow your health club and your health-and-fitness career: your family, your boss, your owner, your community, your employees, and so on. Everyone, either directly or indirectly, is depending on your ability to generate new leads and then turn those leads into new committed customers.

When marketing your health club, you want your message to get out and resonate with your prospects while maintaining consistency. For example, your logo and your catchphrase must remain consistent in your marketing when you change your offer relative to your current marketing campaign. If you want prospective members and current members to know you have the most exclusive health club in the area or you are the most affordable health club within the community, you must repeat that in your message over and over. Use the same consistent message and slogan, but be aware of changing up the offer and hook in your marketing campaigns. For example, if you have the best health club or were voted the number-one health club within your community, make sure that that message is repeated often so people will recognize your club as being number one and get prospects to link that powerful message to your brand.

Get to know your audience and who qualifies as your audience—your targeted demographic. No one can afford to incur wasteful spending. You must take into consideration all aspects of your targets; lifestyles, spending habits, buying patterns, geographical demographics, incomes, and education levels just touch the surface. Naive marketers look primarily at income as being the qualifying factor for membership, but income alone can be very misleading. You probably have your own example of this. Have you ever tried to roll out your own campaign targeting an area labeled "affluent," thinking it was your audience, and yet got a dismal return on your investment? In some cases, enormous income masks enormous debt. These targets with high incomes can't afford to pay attention, much less pay for health-club memberships. You definitely don't want to be in the collection business. Your desired target is consumers with discretionary income, not consumers drowning in debt. Profiling your targets is an absolute must!

MMC® has a research-and-development department that includes a full-time, twenty-four-hours-a-day, seven-days-a-week, 365-days-a-year research center devoted to capturing pertinent information to better serve our clients by profiling their local consumers and prospects. MMC® has been profiling consumers with discretionary income for the sports industry since the late 1980s and best of all, we pay for all the research. As I stated before, we pay all of our own expenses, and profiling the best consumers for our clients happens at our expense.

Establishing a good relationship with your target market is a very important element in positioning your brand and maintaining the desired reputation of your brand in the marketplace. When it comes to brand management, most health clubs are confused as to who is responsible for this position. In reality, every person involved with your club is responsible for your brand management. The marketer is responsible for how your brand is communicated and perceived within the marketplace, while your front-counter person has just as much responsibility because he or she is responsible for the first impression and customer service.

Customer care, starting with answering the phone properly through assisting members and prospects alike when they come into your club, will contribute a lot in building the reputation of your club. It is not only the packaging of the club's marketing campaigns and the pricing structure but also taking time to understand how the prospect and member feels when he or she comes to your club. Are consumers being left alone to fend for themselves, or are they given guidance and good service so they feel welcome as valued members or guests of the club?

To grow your business, you must first know your prospect's core emotional needs and then design your advertisement to target their emotions, not yours. Another great benefit of brand management through superb customer service is that birds of a feather flock together. If your member is health conscious and financially qualified to buy a membership then the odds are good that their friends are as well. If you acquire one member and get him or her committed to a health-club membership, when it comes time for his or her buddies to choose a health club, the buddy will definitely choose your health club because his or her buddy is already in a committed relationship with the club.

By now you know I am a fan of using a lower barrier-to-entry as a hook (the draw) for grabbing the attention of the masses and locking new members up in long-term relationships with our clients' clubs. These introductory memberships can then be upgraded during or after the point of sale. Although, MMC® has numerous other marketing hooks to grow your business that will complement your current business model and achieve your desired results. Lowering the barrier-to-entry is just one hook used in the Cash campaign.

Price can never be your only point of leverage, nor can it ever be presented as the superior part of your health club's product or services. It can be used only as a hook to get the prospects' attention. This is where most owners and operators sink the ship when trying to implement this kind of promotion on their own. All they see is the tip of the iceberg—the initial offer (the hook)—but they fail to see the enormous substance beneath, supporting the tip.

Even when this marketing hook is deployed by MMC®, there is no danger of engaging the undesirable consumer, thanks to MMC®'s vetting system for qualifying prospects. There is also a built-in safeguard to eliminate any undesirables from buying a health-club membership: the club's staff collects all membership revenue and signs all membership agreements. In short, the final decision whether to approve the applicant or not is yours; you maintain full control.

By mastering all media and platforms, MMC®'s team has developed, tested, and successfully implemented a customer-building approach that is unprecedented in the industry today. Specifically, we are able to address the stagnant marketplace by tapping into new segments therefore generating immediate cash, increasing monthly receivables, developing new relationships, and solidifying unparalled member retention. This is not a theory but a proven method, and it's a powerful solution for our participating health clubs.

Our approach involves a loyalty-based relationship that will connect with your market. Today's clubs are faced with at-risk memberships, guest fees, and revenues from juice bars, pro shops, tanning salons, personal-training sessions, and so on, which has been contributed to the current economic climate, lifestyles, and conditioned spending habits of today's consumer. With so many places to train available, customers are leaving their home clubs for discount and bargain memberships. Our research has shown that this group of members account for an average of thirty-five hundred memberships within most markets with populations of twenty-five thousand households or more. Unfortunately, these memberships are divided across multiple health clubs. Marketing to these prospects with coupons, daily deals, and so on only conditions them to wait for the next deal to come along, whether it's from you or your competitor. You can't build long-term relationships and member loyalty in an hour. Relationships require repetition; just like building a muscle, they don't take shape overnight.

MMC®'s model is designed to bring members in on an introductory membership and lock up the long-term relationship (retention is built in) from the beginning. This model gives the club's staff ample time to cultivate the new relationship as opposed to the one-day, five-day, or even one-month passes or month-to-month memberships that dilute the message of health and fitness. I understand these short-term deals are designed to get people through the door to give the sales staff an opportunity to sell the prospects full club memberships, and if the staff is well trained and the prospect is qualified, this marketing concept can be effective. My pushback is there are too many ifs. With MMC®'s Cash campaign, the relationship is already locked up.

The MMC® approach offers a no-risk self-funding solution to execute market-dominating campaigns to grow your loyal customer base. The program start-up requires no cash outlay on the owner's end; MMC® is paid only on performance, and the club owner will handle (and deposit into his or her bank) all of the funds generated. The program is truly no-risk and self-funding, therefore self-propelling. Each phase of the campaign, from the start and moving forward, is propelled and funded by the previous phase. If for any reason the revenue to advance the campaign is not generated, the owner may cancel our agreement at any time without any further financial obligation to MMC®.

MMC® works on a success-only basis, so we receive absolutely no payment unless we are successfully growing your business. MMC® provides the demographic research, market analysis, campaign design and implementation, sales training, coaching, materials, extensive support, consumer profiles, ad copy, ad design, ad layout and a project manager to guide you through every stage of the campaign, eliminating any guesswork and wasteful spending and therefore delivering the desired result: a no-risk self-funding successful member-acquisition marketing campaign targeting the deconditioned segment that grows your club today.

Each project has a unique personality and is custom-designed to meet the needs of the owner or operator. However, it is MMC®'s responsibility to provide a balanced perspective, ensuring that each campaign connects with the local market in a way that can achieve the final goals of the business: to connect with the deconditioned market, engage millennials, rebuild loyalty (as it was in the 1990s), develop unmatched member retention, eliminate discounting memberships, capture higher dollars per membership, and build a sustainable business model for the life of your business.

Since 1991, over 50 percent of our partnering health clubs have raised more than $100,000 in immediate cash; more than 25 percent, over $200,000; more than 10 percent, over $300,000; and numerous clubs, more than $400,000, all in about sixty days or less with our no-risk self-funding health-club Cash campaign. So, when we make the claim that we are the world's leader in health-club marketing, we have the track record to prove it.

Having a great health club to offer your customers is only part of the big picture. Times have changed, and knowing what to do and what not to do is the difference between a campaign that raises $30,000 with no residual income and a marketing campaign that raises $300,000 with increases in back-end revenue by as much as 500 percent. The up-front number (cash collected at the point of sale) is directly proportionate to the residual income you can expect to see from your profit centers: guest fees, personal-training fees, food and beverage revenue, tanning session revenue, and renewal fees. Getting prospects through the door is the challenge of today's owners and operators. Furthermore, getting these prospects to commit to your health club as their exclusive club of choice is an even bigger challenge.

I want to point out once again that I have chosen to use MMC®'s marketing strategy as an example of a sales presentation because it is the very best example I can provide, and since it is designed for owners, it will touch on very important points owners want to have addressed. This is MMC®'s presentation, and you can use our strategy as a template to design your *own* sales presentation for any health-and-fitness product or service. I would be remiss if I didn't share it as well as my five-year marketing plan to grow any health club to ensure you too can design a winning strategy for your products and services.

Most marketers are oblivious to or lack the resources to important components of a successful marketing campaign like demographic research, market analysis, consumer profiling, professional-sales training, data on consumers' buying habits and spending patterns, and so on. It takes in-depth knowledge of all of these areas to maximize your marketing dollars for the greatest ROI while preventing wasteful spending. MMC® knows the power of personalization and has invested in a full-time, twenty-four-hours-a-day, seven-days-a-week research-and-development department that devotes 100 percent of their time to profiling your ideal member. These efforts have produced an unparalleled formula for success by using a variety of campaigns for raising immediate cash, monthly receivables, increasing daily traffic, and planting the seeds for long-term residual income through increased retention around the country. MMC® leaves no stone unturned when it comes to growing your business, and the best part is MMC®'s programs are 100 percent no risk and self-funding!

MMC® has three programs to achieve long-term financial freedom for owners and their businesses:

1. The Cash campaign
2. The EFT campaign
3. The Elite campaign

MMC® also custom-designs six minicampaigns (absolutely free) for our clients to run internally after running MMC®'s Cash campaign. These minicampaigns are specifically designed to capitalize on the increased traffic generated by the Cash campaign and maximize the earning potential of the club's profit centers. By launching these minicampaigns, our clients will begin to condition their members' spending habits.

Giving freebies and bonuses are incredibly valuable tools in building long-term relationships, so invest in caps, gym bags, water bottles, and sweat towels, and start giving out freebies. I practice what I preach, so I have built in numerous added benefits and freebies like the six minicampaigns for the health clubs who chose to partner with MMC®.

MMC®'s three campaigns are scheduled to be launched every year in a specific chronological order, one right after the other, so you'll want to save some of the cash from the initial Cash campaign to fund the second two campaigns. MMC®'s Cash campaign will bring in between $100,000 and $500,000 in immediate cash at the point of sale, as well as hundreds or thousands of new members. This will be your foundation to start building on. During this first year, you will not have the time to launch any of the minicampaigns, nor will you need to. Your primary focus must be on customer service.

The following year, you will want to launch MMC®'s EFT campaign, which will offer a significantly more expensive membership than the introductory membership offered in the Cash campaign. This campaign will focus on raising the perceived value of your club within the marketplace as well as increasing your monthly receivables. The EFT campaign will bring in fewer members than the Cash campaign, so don't expect as huge an influx of members during the second year as you had with the Cash campaign. You will start seeing a slight drop-off in workouts this year, so you will want to compensate for the attrition by running the EFT campaign. The attrition rate will be determined by your previous year's customer service, so do not let up on customer-care programs. This second year, you will launch one to two of the internal low to no-cost minicampaigns to increase revenue in one or two of your profit centers.

The third year, you will launch the Elite campaign, targeting a wealthier demographic with a much higher price-point, again increasing the perceived value of your membership within your market. You will also run one to two more minicampaigns for one or two more profit centers. The Elite campaign will bring in far fewer members than the Cash and EFT campaigns but will cost far less since the population of this demographic is much smaller. MMC®'s Elite campaign is designed to increase the value of a club's brand. This campaign is not a huge moneymaker but will pay for itself tenfold.

Here is what I mean: After the third year, the introductory memberships will be coming up for renewal. If you have done everything right and the economy hasn't gotten worse, you can raise your membership rates to a fair market value because you have been slowly increasing the club's perceived value within the marketplace over the past two to three years. If for some reason the economic climate hasn't changed, you can run another Cash campaign, raising the price-point of the introductory membership, and start the cycle over but with an increased perceived value within the marketplace. You will never offer the original price-point again, because you never want the market to perceive you as a $100, $200, or even $300 club. You want to be perceived as a club of value and great customer service where your members get results, not for offering a cheap membership.

The worst thing you can do is take this price-point and run it year after year or, just as bad, run it on a very limited basis and not maximize its potential. It's like giving a patient the prescribed dosage of a medicine. Too much will result in an overdose and not enough is just as bad as not doing anything at all. The proper dosage is required if you want the patient to overcome the illness. Once you've made the decision, don't try to put the medicine back in the syringe. Go for it; there's no reason for you to stop and pull back. Just enjoy the ride, and build on the momentum. Do not use MMC®'s marketing concept as a business model; use it as a *tool.*

MMC® has had clubs stop the Cash campaign after bringing in five hundred members or so only to regret their decisions to not go deeper into the campaign within just a few short months. Stopping early is a huge mistake; you'll never get another chance to build off the momentum once it is gone. MMC®'s Cash campaign is designed to bring in the masses, and it only makes sense when targeting the deconditioned market and the goal is volume from the beginning. Then and only then will the business have the surplus of members necessary to raise membership rates without worrying about the attrition rate.

This exciting new membership program will substantially enhance your ability to provide current members with an even greater value than ever before. This program involves a very aggressive membership-growth initiative. It is important to note that this new program offers a membership opportunity far different from anything you have provided in the past and, as such, is not directly comparable to the membership plans to which you are accustomed. We believe you will be incredibly excited about this one-time offer, as this new membership category is specifically designed for the casual members in your community, which will provide the greatest value your club will ever offer. However, there are dramatic differences between your premium (platinum) membership and this introductory membership, so there is no reason to worry your existing members may migrate to the introductory membership offer.

MMC®'s Cash campaign is designed to be launched in four phases:

We start with a soft internal launch with signs in the club and e-mails to present and past members. The revenue collected from this soft launch is then used to seed the direct-mail campaign. During this time, MMC®'s staff is pulling all of the demographic data, compiling the data for the profiling process, studying the competitive overview, creating ad copy and design, training your staff, and so on in preparation for the external launch.

The second phase is some local newspaper and radio ads. Although these media are dying, they still have some listeners and readers who are health and fitness conscious. A campaign like ours is based on guerilla marketing, and you must not leave one stone unturned. These delivery systems are especially important for getting the word-of-mouth marketing started.

The third phase is the driving force of the campaign; direct mail will be deployed through four consecutive mail drops to profile targets selected by a criteria-based formula. This is the most important phase of the campaign. This entire campaign has been designed around targeting the deconditioned market to balance out the membership base while increasing revenue through all profit centers. If you are not 100 percent committed to this phase of the campaign *do not embark on this campaign* because you will just deplete your core customers and ruin your business. The success of this phase is based on the profile, if you do not have access to the profile and lack the proper tools to engage the deconditioned market, do not attempt to run (ruin) this campaign. Each week's direct mail launch is determined and propelled by the previous week's intake of revenue. So, at no time is the owner at risk or out of pocket to fund the direct mail.

FYI, mailing lists can be compiled from thousands of different sources for thousands of different list profiles. Lists are available for individuals, organizations, and for businesses. With individuals, there are a tremendous number of choices available, such as average household income, head-of-household age, type of home, date the home was built, date the home was last sold and for how much, home value, mortgage holders, families with children living at home, number of occupants in the household, number of occupants under the age of eighteen, genders, hobbies, interests, sports played, magazine subscriptions bought, donor activities, mail-order buyers, credit-card purchases, and many, many other options, making the choices in lists virtually limitless.

Some of the most common ways business lists can be generated are by number of employees, amount of annual sales, type of business, branch or home office locations, contact names, and many other various segments. MMC® pulls hundreds of lists and combine multiple lists to identify qualified consumers who fit our profile, specifically designed to target the deconditioned segment, based on geographic, demographic, and psychographic data.

MMC® has tried literally thousands of lists from numerous list companies, and then tracked those results. Besides tracking, we need to know what works best (gets the best responses), we also want to track what generates the very best type of business (the most revenue, the best prospects, and so on) and what gives us the very best ROI for our marketing dollars. This ROI is learned through mistakes and successes, which MMC® has experienced for you so you don't suffer the disappointments and losses. The key is to track all of the results, not just the responses. Just like many things in life, you get better at something the more you do it, the more information you have, and the more you understand what works and what doesn't.

The fourth and final phase of our Cash campaign is the closeout. This is when all media and platforms are enlisted. We leave no stone unturned. You can easily raise 20 percent of the total gross of the campaign in the last two weeks when the closeout is managed properly. Again, the campaign is set up this way with built-in adjusters to accommodate the circumstances. If the client has reached the desired results before the closeout, the client can choose to do a soft, quiet closeout; if the client is short of the desired result, the client can push the closeout as hard as necessary to achieve the desired result. Either way, the closeout is extremely important because not only do you lock up all of the last-minute procrastinators but you also inform the community that this once in a lifetime opportunity is coming to a close and will never be offered again. This announcement helps you get back to your normal pricing. In addition, it gives you a "real" reason why you can no longer offer the introductory membership since you are under contractual agreement with a company in Florida that specializes in fitness awareness programs and they are the driving force behind this campaign. You can honestly say your rates have always been X and this was just a campaign designed and managed by MMC® to bring community awareness to health-and-fitness.

The next step is forward thinking. Now, that the owner has raised some cash, paid the bills, and put some money in the bank and a little in his or her pocket, he or she can start preparing for the future growth of the business by starting with MMC®'s EFT campaign.

Our EFT (electronic funds transfer or monthly receivables) campaign is designed to raise our clients' monthly receivables. After closing out MMC®'s Cash campaign our clients are not looking to raise quick cash, since they ran our Cash campaign the previous year, but they would love to add to their current membership base. The EFT campaign is designed for exactly that. Instead of advertising a PIF membership, we offer a monthly payment model, although we can incorporate a PIF option for those clubs who wish to raise a little more cash as well. MMC® has also designed a three-tier membership for our EFT campaign, just as we have for our Cash campaign. It is extremely important to stay consistent with your marketing message and model.

The following year, the club should launch MMC®'s Elite campaign. This campaign targets the affluent demographic with discretionary income through demographic profiling and select consumer spending. MMC®'s staff will consult with you and custom-design a marketing campaign around your current business model, membership rates and budget. This campaign is designed to attract consumers where cost and inconvenience can be overcome by the prestige of belonging to and having the best. Because there are far fewer consumers who fall into this category, you can expect to have far fewer prospects; all things are relative. This platinum membership is the full, all-inclusive membership you may currently have in place today. MMC®'s team will just dress it up, make it more attractive, more desirable and therefore, more sellable.

By the time you launch the Elite campaign you will be in your third year of the five-year model. The fourth and fifth years the club owner will launch the remaining minicampaigns taking the business through the five-year model. These minicampaigns will require very little if any, investment but will pay huge dividends over the life of your business. These are the kind of programs most managers know how to create and develop, but in most cases, can rarely find the time to do so.

Now that the club has brought in all of these new members after running MMC®'s Cash campaign, the staff will be spending far more of their time cultivating relationships and will have even less time to devote to marketing. With our program, you and your staff won't have to worry about marketing to grow your business because we will be focused on it for you. These minicampaigns will be 100 percent turnkey, and you will not pay MMC® an additional dime for them. They are our gift to you, your staff, and your members for letting us be a part of the experience.

Clubs should always start with the Cash campaign to raise revenue, even if cash is not an issue. All health clubs have debt that needs to be paid or equipment leases that can be paid off to ease the financial burden that is hindering the business' growth. Besides, you'll need cash to support the other two campaigns. Every business should have at least a five-year marketing plan to guarantee the growth of the club, and this is why I have structured this model to grow any club for a minimum of five years. Every health club should have at least six different marketing campaigns designed and ready to launch at any time. With six campaigns, you will have your marketing strategy prepared for the next two to three years.

With just a little bit of thought, it is easy to take the same old products or services and spin them in a different light. As a marketer, you must have a strategy and always be ready to launch a campaign in a moment's notice. Be creative. You do not have to change your business; all you have to do is make it more appealing to more people. Since I started working as a consultant in the mid-1980s, it has been challenging to get owners and managers to commit to marketing strategies that will carry them throughout the year much less over the next five years. Ninety percent of the time, they are so happy with the cash collected they forget about the pain that got them to call me in the first place.

MMC®'s Cash campaign's supremacy over any campaign ever designed for the health-and-fitness industry goes unchallenged. Most clubs—and marketing companies, for that matter—would never be able to afford, have the resources or personnel to launch this mammoth campaign. Never in most club's history or future would the club have the opportunity to knock on deconditioned prospects' door in their immediate areas and deliver their clubs' messages completely uninterrupted. MMC® has made it possible because our campaigns completely pay for themselves and our team performs 99 percent of the work behind the scenes; that is why I say MMC® is health-club marketing on steroids. Our clients' health clubs get bigger and stronger within just sixty days.

The Cash campaign was never meant to be a business model; it is simply meant to be a marketing campaign that takes a club through the difficult times or slow seasons and puts the business into a position where an owner can engage and acquire more members but at a much higher price-point in the future. In most cases, if you are able to capture the largest part of the market, or dominate your market, the first time, then you can get right back to the club's rack-rate membership a lot faster, and you won't need to run the Cash campaign ever again. Once you have established your rates and your perceived value within your community, you can do smaller-scale campaigns to sustain the growth you've already achieved. Then, you can increase your membership rates to whatever your market will bear.

Always guard against the downside. The only possible downside to MMC®'s Cash campaign would be inexperience, incompetence, or laziness. The campaign can't fail; only the human components can. This is not the type of campaign you let an amateur hack at to see whether he or she can get the ball close to the pin or inside the leather (a golf analogy). These innovative health-club marketing campaigns require a team of marketing professionals who are up to par with relevant data and have experienced in growing businesses. There is a bright future for the industry, but clubs must increase rates and abandon the $9.99 model. Health-club memberships for just fitness should cost a minimum of $30.00–$60.00 per month to ensure a sustainable business model for growth and customer care. It's time for a new paradigm.

Twenty-five years ago, I set out to bring affordable health and fitness to all Americans, and I certainly accomplished that goal. Whether affordable health-club memberships have been a direct or indirect result of my campaigns, intentionally or inadvertently, the goal was realized just the same. The Cash campaign I designed in the late 1980s changed the industry's model of selling memberships by lowering the barrier-to-entry. Millions upon millions of Americans can now purchase health-club memberships for as low as $99.00 per year or $9.99 per month.

The low barrier-to-entry marketing concept is a win-win; it is a hook for businesses to grab the attention of the consumers who have not been properly engaged. This introductory membership allows the new member limited access to the fitness floor and all other amenities, products, and services are à la carte. Health clubs are a business and must make money as well as be profitable to motivate owners to stay in business. These introductory members pay lower membership fees, and for getting such a great value, they agree to work out during the club's slow times of the day or slow seasons. They choose to adjust their schedules accordingly and have the option to stay in the introductory membership category or upgrade to a full club membership, either at the point of sale or anytime during the term of their membership. They pay extra for any extra products or services they choose to buy.

With this membership category, health and fitness is affordable for all Americans and profitable for all club owners. Owners are filling in dead times of the day with members who will spend in the profit centers, and consumers get a great introductory rate. This concept (a low barrier-to-entry) will not be successful if it is targeting the health-conscious market. This campaign is designed specifically for the untapped segments of the market and MMC® is the only company with the formula. There is an old Chinese saying that goes something like this; if you handle a master carpenter's tools, be prepare to hurt yourself.

Touching people's lives in a positive way has been extremely rewarding for me over the years. Exercise, proper eating habits, and plenty of uninterrupted sleep are the triad for a long, happy, healthy life. MMC®'s Cash, EFT, and Elite campaigns are the triad for the financial health of a club. I am so proud and grateful I was able to help millions of people change their lives by making joining health clubs affordable. My life changed for the better the day I walked into that first health club in Nashville, Tennessee in 1982, and I hope after reading this book your life too will change for the better.

Wishing you good health and prosperity,
Chuck Thompson

PS. Please take a few minutes and write a review for my book and post it on as many websites and platforms as possible, with a direct link to where your friends and followers can buy *Affordable Health and Fitness: The Business of Health and Fitness,* and be sure to register with my company and personal websites www.mmctoday.com, www.healthclubmarketingmmc.com and www.chuckthompson. guru (not dot com) for freebies and updates. If you wish to contact us at MMC®, you may call 904-217-3762; toll free 877-620-8135 or e-mail me at chuck@mmctoday.com. For comments or any other correspondence, please use my personal address at chuck@chuck-thompson.guru (not dot com).

Thank you.

Mulligan:
A mulligan is when a golfer or business gets a second chance to take another shot whether it's a shot at a pin to improve the golfer's score or a health club getting another shot at growing their business with no penalty—a "do-over." (Chuck Thompson)
MMC® has a mulligan for growing your business today.
Mulligan Marketing Concepts® Since 1991
Office: 904-217-3762
Toll Free: 877-620-8135
www.healthclubmarketingmmc.com
www.mmctoday.com
chuck@mmctoday.com
chuck@chuckthompson.guru (not dot com)

Made in the USA
Lexington, KY
10 September 2017